The Hypnotic Use of Waking Dreams

Exploring Near-Death Experiences

without the Flatlines

Paul W. Schenk PsyD

Crown House Publishing Limited

www.crownhouse.co.uk

First published by

Crown House Publishing Ltd
Crown Buildings, Bancyfelin, Carmarthen, Wales, SA33 5ND, UK
www.crownhouse.co.uk

and

Crown House Publishing Company LLC
6 Trowbridge Drive, Suite 5, Bethel, CT 06801-2858, USA
www.CHPUS.com

Copyright © 2006 by Paul W. Schenk PsyD

ISBN 10: 1845900308

ISBN 13: 978-1845900304

LCCN: 2006929712

Printed in the UK by
Cromwell Press, Trowbridge, Wiltshire

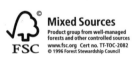

Mixed Sources
Product group from well-managed
forests and other controlled sources
www.fsc.org Cert no. TT-TOC-2082
© 1996 Forest Stewardship Council
FSC

Contents

Foreword

Dr. Paul Schenk is a skilled and sensitive therapist who has had the courage—and the kindness—to integrate the spiritual dimension of life into his therapy. This is important, because early in the 21st century tens of millions of baby boomers are waking up to their own, inner spiritual callings. Therefore, *The Hypnotic Use of Waking Dreams: Exploring Near-Death Experiences without the Flatlines* is a timely book and one that is destined to be helpful to many readers. There are a lot of people now, as I know from my own work, who are almost desperate, trying to make sense of the emerging feelings and spiritual strivings that naturally accompany mid-life.

The trouble is, there are many "professionals" out there who are willing to step in and offer these people pat answers, which may make them feel great at first—but only for a little while. Dr. Schenk's approach is different; it is well-grounded in psychological knowledge and tempered with his true excellence as a practitioner. (I know, because I have watched him work.) He appreciates the reality that spiritual progress is a difficult challenge that does not yield to simplistic formulas.

So, this fine work is not another platitude-filled New Age book about dreams, near-death experiences, or reincarnation. Instead, it is a gripping chronicle of ordinary people's adventures in exploring a vitally important, but mostly subterranean, dimension of the mind. The book relates case after riveting case of people who, under Dr. Schenk's guidance and with his support, have plumbed parts of themselves that are not normally accessible to awareness. These case studies certainly are page-turners, to say the least. Yet, the deeper message of the book is that these abilities lie within all of us and are easier to access than we usually imagine.

As Dr. Schenk says, the world has been enthralled by near-death experiences since 1975. Those who almost died but are revived tell us that a light-filled world of love, joy, and peace lies just over the horizon of physical death. They say that they learn from their experiences that the most important thing we can do, while alive in this world, is to learn to love. Hence, if there were some way to have near-death experiences or similar experiences while we are still alive—and safely, of course!—it is not unreasonable to imagine that this discovery would advance the cause of higher civilization. I think that this is the most exciting prospect that Dr. Schenk's work offers. It is wonderful and inspiring that he has been able to tap into important, forgotten realms of the mind by straightforward and comprehensible techniques.

This is a pioneering work. Dr. Schenk is in the vanguard of an emerging, inexorable movement that acknowledges the central position of the spirit in human affairs. And it is a fine thing that he has done this while remaining strictly within the parameters of reason and sound clinical practice. I have already recommended this book to several psychotherapists-in-training who want to integrate spiritual counseling into their practices. I believe that Dr. Schenk's book will continue to inspire therapists and spiritual seekers in the future.

Raymond A. Moody, Jr., M.D.
Author of *Life After Life*
Anniston, AL

Preface

Since Raymond Moody published *Life after Life* in 1975, the popular press has responded to the public's fascination with near-death experiences (NDEs) with a variety of books. For the interested reader, please refer to the bibliography for some suggested reading. As one author noted, "NDEs are probably the most direct kind of experiential knowledge about the after death state we can have: they are certainly the most emotionally and intellectually powerful kinds of knowledge that, in some form, we survive death, *for those who experience them.*"[1] But as another author reminds us, "Reading or hearing about [an NDE] is very different from having one, simply because they are indescribable even in metaphor, the language of Spirit."[2] The logical extension of this is easy to describe:

> … it would be quite helpful if we each personally had an NDE, but after an extensive study of NDE[s], I don't recommend that. The near part of an NDE is too tricky! Most people who come that near to death do not give us an interesting report of what happened afterwards; they get buried![3]

In this book, I will share with you some of the profound experiences and insights my clients have reported while using hypnosis to dream *during* therapy. Therapists have made use of clients' dreams since the days of Freud, but we usually rely on the fragments of the dream that the person can remember days later during the therapy session. By having my clients dream during the therapy session in what I call a *waking dream*, they and I are able to work with the content and emotion of the dream in real time. These dreams differ from ordinary dreams in that *clients always experience themselves as someone else in a waking dream*. Throughout the book, I will refer to this someone else as the "dream character".

The setting for the dream inevitably involves a different place and time, and often a change in gender. Unlike nighttime dreams, however, the final stage of a waking dream typically includes the death of the dream character. This is why it is critical that clients are never themselves in these dreams. I will not risk the emotional impact of intentionally taking someone through his or her own death in a dream! What happens *after* the death experience of the dream character is a major focus of this book.

Chapter 1 introduces you to the concept of waking dreams and describes seven ways they can be used to help people resolve a variety of personal problems, enhance their intuitive abilities, and enrich the spiritual aspect of their lives.

Chapter 2 begins with a review of what has been reported in the literature for more than thirty years on the phenomenon of near-death experiences. These phenomena are then discussed in the context of what occurs in the final stage of a waking dream.

Chapter 3 describes the prototype of a waking dream. Just as many NDEs do not include all of the core components of a prototypical NDE, few waking dreams completely match the prototype. However, because they occur by choice, it is helpful to have a good understanding of the many forms waking dreams can take. This enhances the opportunities for using them both with more confidence and greater effectiveness.

Chapters 4 through 7 present a variety of actual waking dreams with detailed case transcripts. These serve to demonstrate some of the many ways that waking dreams can be used to facilitate personal, even transpersonal, change.

Chapters 8 and 9 explore the parallels between waking dreams and past-life therapy. In many parts of the world, people believe that the soul experiences hundreds of lifetimes, each of which affords opportunities for learning. Past-life therapy extends the notion that current problems sometimes have their origins in past events by looking to other lifetimes when the events of the current lifetime are insufficient to account for the current problem. For example, there is considerable anecdotal research that many phobias resolve quickly with past-life therapy.

Chapters 10 and 11 use additional transcripts from waking dreams to probe some of the spiritual implications this work can have for each of us.

In the final chapter, I summarize and synthesize the other chapters with a discussion of some of the spiritual, soul-level implications that have emerged for both my clients and me from this work.

Paul W. Schenk

Chapter 1
The Things You Can Do with a Good Dream

When I died I had an overwhelming experience of calm and peace. I was floating above the ocean and felt absolute harmony with everything around me.

The light is so bright. I feel like I'm floating. There is a lot of loving presence here.

My parents are worried about the ship sinking, about the storm. They just woke me up. We're leaving the cabin. People are running. My mother and I lost my dad in the crowd. I'm off the ship now. I seem to be floating up in the air. My mother is next to me, we must have died. We fell into the cold water getting into the lifeboat. I can see my body sinking in the ocean. I was trying to touch my body, but it was too far away and everyone disappeared. [*Pause.*] My grandmother is there! She took my hand! Now she's guiding me, telling me to come with her. Mom's up there with her. I see the Light now, a big sun. I'm so happy to be with my grandmother again!

When I died I saw my funeral ... Then I proceeded to float up and I found my wife. She was very excited to see me. I had an overwhelming experience of feeling loved. All of my sad thoughts had left me and I just filled up with happy ones.

If you have previously read about near-death experiences, these descriptions will have a familiar ring to them. For more than three decades now, researchers have provided us with fascinating glimpses of life-after-life that sometimes occur in individuals following a heart attack or other life-threatening crisis. Triggered by potentially fatal situations, survivors report incredible tranquility and peacefulness as they float out of the physical body into an intensely bright light where they are typically greeted lovingly by others: deceased relatives, spirit guides, angels, religious figures, etc. When the experience lasts long enough, these survivors engage

1

in a non-judgmental life review often accompanied by significant insights. Despite the fact that the experience is over in a matter of seconds, most report profound, durable, life-altering aftereffects of a positive nature.

The descriptions above are not from people who have suffered a close call with death, however. What they are describing took place in my office during psychotherapy sessions. Unlike traditional near-death experiences in which the heart often stops, these people were in no distress. They were all sitting or lying comfortably on my couch.

Waking dreams provide a vehicle that enables people to experience many of the phenomena associated with a true near-death experience, but without any of the life-threatening risks. The varied case studies that follow, with their extensive transcripts of actual waking dreams, demonstrate a variety of ways that I have used waking dreams to help people resolve problems ranging from the specific to the existential. Transcripts, of course, are limited in their ability to convey the emotional richness that is so integral to the experience. Nonetheless, as you read each of the case studies, I hope you will increasingly sense the transformative potential of waking dreams.

Aided by straightforward hypnotic techniques, my clients experience vivid dream-like imagery during the psychotherapy session in which they become the main character in a fictional life. The life of the dream character may include insightful parallels to the client's own life, such as Dorothy experienced in *The Wizard of Oz*, but the true power of the waking dream typically begins when the dream character dies. At this transitional moment, clients typically report the first of many of the characteristics associated with a true near-death experience. Floating out of the body of the dream character and into the Light, most clients meet what they describe as spirit guides or other non-physical beings whose function seems to replicate that of the figures who present in a true NDE.

Among other things, waking dreams usually include a non-judgmental life review, an opportunity to release faulty beliefs and feelings of guilt, reunion with loved ones, and transforming experiences of being loved unconditionally. Unlike a true NDE, an important part of this experience is a meeting between the dream character and the client in which the dream character offers the client support and guidance for his or her own life struggles. The process often concludes with an assurance that the guides and/or the dream character will remain available to the client in an ongoing relationship, assisting, coaching, and supporting the client's efforts to change.

Throughout the book, I refer to these after-death beings as "spirit guides" or simply "guides". In doing so, I wish to be pragmatic without being presumptive. It is certainly possible that these guides are merely creations of the client's imagination, just like the dream character and others who appear in the waking dream. Because both their function and the emotional responses that their presence elicits seem analogous to similar encounters described in true NDEs, I chose a label descriptive of that function.

Waking dreams allow people to work on a variety of issues:

1. Sometimes they discover previously unrecognized faulty assumptions about a problem.

Once identified, these faulty beliefs fall away. As this happens, new solutions quickly emerge. Consider the example of Matthew who had long perceived power as a kind of magic that only women have. The only way he could have power, therefore, was to be in a relationship with a woman. As a result, he became depressed and anxious whenever he was in between relationships. In one of his waking dreams, he saw himself as a young girl, Antoinette, who spent the rest of her life in a convent as a nun. By the time of her death, she had become the Mother Superior. Comparing the characters in the waking dream with his own life, Matthew noted:

> When you asked me to look for people in the nun's life, I realized I couldn't ... I knew the father in the girl's story was a parent in my life, but I didn't know which one. Still don't. But then I had a set of thoughts that went, "Oh, if it's my father, and he really had this kind of power, what I saw then was a man who was so afraid of how he would misuse power that he wasn't going to let himself have any." And that's stupid. Power is just another form of magic. You don't have to be consumed by it. It's another form of energy. It's not that big a deal.

3

What she [*Antoinette*] saw earlier was—it's a kinesthetic experience, how the hell do I put it into words ... okay, "Magic is external to me. You go out of yourself towards it, grab something outside of yourself, and try to get incorporated *by* it." She found that God has to subtract from Himself to create an emptiness into which the magic can enter. The cabalistic statement is, "God created nothing in order for there to be a space into which He could enter." God subtracted from Himself. What she got was a kinesthetic of, "You let God into you. That creates a space into which the magic enters." The magic is an energy exchange between you and God—to be prosaic about it. [*I interjected*, "Did, you get that in a kinesthetic way?"] Oh, yea. Oh, yea. I was flooded with light.

Then, a minute later, he found another faulty assumption. In the waking dream, the young girl had gone through a period of intense loneliness as a teenager in the convent.

That was the shift in me about . . . Ahhh! This is relevant actually. Two years ago, a woman told me something which I heard, and knew she was absolutely right, but didn't know what to do with it. She said that I confused loneliness with missing God.

The nun had the experience (of the loneliness) which is why I said I thought I was in exile. I thought I was like being put in "time out," and *He* has to take me out of time out. It's only a separation. I got it. ... Oh! He's been waiting for me to come back!

2. People can safely try out a new solution in the virtual reality of the waking dream, modifying it as needed.

As an analogy, consider the main concept of the 1993 movie *Groundhog Day* happening in a trance-induced virtual reality. In the movie, the main character finds himself trapped in a 24-hour time loop. Every day when he awakes it is the same calendar day. Each day he experiments with different ways of resolving his problems, drawing on his successes and failures from the previous attempts. When he finally works out a solution he truly likes, he gets out of the time loop.

One client, a middle-aged professional woman, Emily, was wrestling with whether to risk shifting the focus of her work to an area that held much more appeal for her, but that might alienate her from much of the conservative community where she lived. In one of her waking dreams, she was a professor, Winston, and the administrator of a seminary. As the dream went on, she narrated:

> I've called in another one of the professors, Gilbert, because of pressure from influential parents of some of the students. The parents are complaining that this professor has been filling their sons' heads with things they don't want them to think about. He is questioning and promoting questioning in the students. He is arguing with me because he knows from our prior conversations that I agree with him. But I don't give in. I tell him if he doesn't stop, I'll let him go. These people are too important. They give too much money to us. I can't ignore them. His reaction is surprising, because he looks at me with sadness, almost pity. I'm embarrassed and furious. He leaves, and soon after leaves the seminary.

> I find it ironic: the seminary continues to struggle and yet he prospers. Gilbert starts his own small school. Only the brightest, most open-minded students seek him out. Even though he doesn't have the most money, he still seems to prosper. Meanwhile, I don't grow and the seminary doesn't grow. I realize too late there was nothing else in my life, so I retire from the seminary on a small pension. I'm very bored and bitter, and I feel like I sold it all. I just sold out my life. I sold my potential for financial security, but all I bought was boredom.

Soon after this comment in her narration of the waking dream, Winston died. Following his death, I invited Emily to revisit the decision Winston had made that day in the seminary office when he and Gilbert had argued. I suggested she implement an alternative decision and notice what difference it made.

> It was not very satisfying to have power over sheep. I have to learn to be true to myself. (If I changed the decision) I'd leave the seminary with Gilbert and start a new one. In that setting I see myself having a challenging, vibrant life, growing and learning and teaching. We took a lot of financial risk—and social risk. We're very unpopular with the majority of the people, just as he really was. But the best and brightest learned from him and would have learned from me, too. They soak in knowledge like a sponge, never depleting mine but enhancing it, teaching me in return.

Now, five years since that waking dream, Emily is well into the transition in her own work. She is still valued by her traditional

5

referral sources despite having become much more open in her pursuit of this new direction in her career. The fear and apprehension that had plagued her for some time have gradually abated as she has given herself permission to pursue her true interests.

3. In waking dreams, people can develop abilities and relationship skills they currently lack.

A recently divorced woman, Donna, brought her two children to see me for some help dealing with the fallout from the breakup of the family. In one of her individual sessions, she had a waking dream in which she was the wife of a Southern plantation owner in the pre-Civil War period. In her dream, Donna's husband had died young and left her with two children to raise and a plantation to manage. As she explored the remainder of Donna's life in the dream, she experienced the confidence and competent manner in which she managed the plantation. She noted with some humor that the other plantation owners in the community, all men, did not take kindly to the undeniable truth that she was more successful than they were. Following her death in that dream, Donna had a strong sense that her own two children were with her to help her remain aware of her own competency as she deals with the stereotyped expectations of some of her professional colleagues in the traditionally male-dominated field in which she works.

4. Sometimes in a waking dream people experience a problem from an opposing perspective.

This is particularly helpful for clients who have felt "victimized" in some way by life. Emily (see number 2) had not only been looking to move in a new direction professionally, she had also remained somewhat "stuck" following the death of her long-term partner. Previously, she had experienced a number of other losses in her life. In her grieving over her partner's death, she wrestled with the unfairness that she always seemed to be the one who was left behind. In one of her waking dreams, her partner appeared in the role of a spouse. In Emily's role as the dream character, this time she was the first of them to die. Floating in the Light, she decided that it was no easier to be the first to die than to be the one left behind.

6

She had had to deal with other losses as well. As the owner of a small business, Emily had suffered quite a financial loss when a trusted employee embezzled funds. She experienced the other side of this relationship in another waking dream in which Emily saw herself as a young man, Clark, who wanted to join the military. In the dream, his mother was opposed to this. Over a period of about twenty minutes, she related the following events in her dream:

> My mother inherited some money from her parents and sent me away. She shouldn't have done that. She couldn't make me go, but bribed me with money to go and find another type of work. She wants me to go to other countries and export things back to our country. The money is a temptation and I take it, but I don't look into anything productive. It is my first time out from under her watchful eye, and I have a good time [*smiling*]. I drink a lot, go to whore houses, become friends with seedy people. I'm just too naive to know they're around just for the money. I don't know much about the world . . . I'm sick. I have no money left. All of my companions that I thought were friends are gone. I'm homeless. A lady finds me and takes me in. She feeds me, and nurses me back to health. She has an apothecary shop. She tells me I can work in it. She teaches me what the different herbs and roots and teas do. Once again I abuse the power she gives me. I find out which ones make you feel good and I start taking them. I become addicted. She has to make me leave. I'm homeless again. This time the illness is from withdrawal . . . I get on a ship and hide. I'm dying. What a waste. I didn't have enough courage to do what I wanted to do. I never connected with anyone. I used two very good opportunities and destroyed myself with them, and hurt the people who were trying to help me.

Following Clark's death, I suggested Emily do a life review and notice what she learned from this "wasted life".

> I have to learn to give as well as to take. I was supposed to learn that but I didn't. It was too easy and felt too good to take. It was too much work to give anything back. I also learned that I need people—real connections with people, not superficial but real. Love is much more important than feeling good.

> I tell myself, "Now you've got to come back as the people being hurt because you have to learn what that's like. Learn what it's like to be on the other side."

Subsequent to this waking dream, Emily's anger at the employee who had embezzled from her subsided considerably, and continued to abate in the months that followed. She still pursued legal avenues to the situation, but was able to do so from a much calmer perspective.

5. Once a new solution is clear, many clients establish a cue based on the waking dream that serves as a self-generated reminder to use the new solution when that particular situation occurs again.

One woman, Jane, generated the idea of hearing her dream character whisper "purple" in her ear whenever she began acting jealous around friends or colleagues. While I monitored this over the next several months, she reported that not only had she heard "purple" on a number of occasions (reaffirming how much of a problem this behavior had been), but that many of her friends had commented on the positive shift in her interactions where jealousy was concerned.

6. Clients develop new insights into current relationships based on relationships between the characters in the dream.

In one waking dream, a young woman, Betsy, saw herself as an old man, Stephen, sitting on a park bench. His wife had died, and he had no contact with his two grown sons.

> I never really got along with them. I have money and don't know what to do with it. I don't want to give it to my sons.

Betsy noted that Stephen seemed very resentful. She said, "He was just disappointed. Nothing went the way he wanted." Following his death, she reported the following discussion with him:

> He's telling me to do something with my life. Don't be like he was. He's very sad now. He's crying. He wasn't very nice. He never gave time for anyone. He was very selfish. He realizes this now.
>
> He was the middle of three children. He didn't really get along with his brother and younger sister. He never really connected with his mom and dad. Both parents died when he was 17. He moved out and started on his own. He never kept in touch with his brother and

sister. He lost a bunny when he was little. He loved that bunny. He put all his love in that bunny and it died. He didn't care for anyone else after that. He tried to love his wife; she just got annoying.

He's telling me to love as many people as possible. It is sad when you go to your funeral and no one is there except your sons—out of obligation. He's telling me to call all my brothers and sisters and tell them how much I love them.

I suggested that Betsy ask Stephen what he would have to give up to let go of feeling so unlovable. He told her he would have to let go of his pride. Given the choice between being proud and alone or risking love, Stephen accepted my invitation to have his wife join him there in the Light. The client then reported:

She's very happy to see him. He's shocked! He thought she hated him.

I suggested that Betsy allow herself to experience this firsthand instead of from the third-person perspective. She continued:

I'm very happy. It's a nice feeling. She loves me, she really loves me. Someone really loves me!

I then invited Stephen's parents to join him. Smiling, Betsy continued:

There they are! They're hugging me. They love me, too!

As we explored metaphorical connections between the dream characters and people in her own life, Betsy reported a number of parallels like those found in *The Wizard of Oz*. Stephen's parents were representative of Betsy's aunt and uncle; Stephen's aunt and uncle were representative of her own parents. When Stephen was a child, these relatives had been nice to him, but had moved away and he had missed them. There were more connections. His wife in the dream was a parallel to one of the Betsy's grandmothers. His two sons in the dream were a parallel to two of Betsy's sisters. Two more of her siblings were represented by Stephen's brother and sister. Finally, a teenage girl whom Stephen had befriended as an old man in his neighborhood had personality traits of one of Betsy's nieces.

As Betsy ended the dialogue with him in this waking dream, I asked if he had any other messages for her about all these people gathering together there in the Light with him. He told her:

> Stay in contact. Why? Because they love you.

Not only did the dream provide Betsy with an intense experience of feeling loved by so many people, it also let her experience the consequences of the alternative in the form of the lonely, bitter man sitting on the park bench. Notice how the dream took advantage of many different relationships from Stephen's life, bringing the essence of those people into many different relationships in Betsy's own life. Love is not just between soul mates. It is a feeling we experience internally that can arise from any relationship we nurture.

7. Clients often explore metaphysical, existential, or spiritual issues in waking dreams, typically following the death of the dream character.

One of Emily's (see number 4) other waking dreams provides an example of this. In this dream, she is a young woman, Tarea, who grew up in a gypsy community in Europe in the 1800s. At age 16, she became pregnant by her mother's boyfriend who subsequently left. She gave birth to a son who became very special to her: "I never cared so much about anybody." One day when her son was four years old, men on horseback rode through the camp to run them out of the area. Her son ran out to see what was happening and was killed by one of the horses. Until she died some 25 years later, she never let anyone get close to her again (despite the efforts of several people who sought to help) because, as she said, "It hurts too much." On her deathbed, Tarea laid waiting for the darkness to come, but instead she said the Light came. With it came understanding:

> I blew it. I know now that no matter how bad it hurts, it's all worth it. Love. I just wasted so much. I'm going to have to do that one again.

> People tried to comfort me, tried to help me. They tried to get close to me sometimes. But I never allowed it.

I suggested Tarea and Emily meet and talk with each other.

> It's all worth it. That's what she's sharing with me now. That's why she came back. She says to never close the door. It's too hard to re-open it.

We worked with the metaphor of the door as Emily had experienced it emotionally in her own life.

> That's a scary thought to take it down; then you can't close it.

Asked about the benefits of keeping the door open or taking it down, Emily remarked:

> (It's about) understanding more about love, purpose, all of it. It's like being on the other side, millions of tiny sparkles. It's wonderful. It's not something that can be put into words. It's so beautiful! It's not scary here. What's scary is what I have to go through to get here.

> It's all worth it. Everything is worth it … You have to receive if you give it. You always get back … If it was easy, if it was all easy, there wouldn't be much point. How could I learn if it was all easy?

This last point routinely becomes a gateway to what is often one of the most significant aspects of the therapy process. I believe our culture continues to value an emphasis on the five senses at the expense of an additional way of knowing: our intuitive sense. Facilitated by the guides and dream characters in a series of waking dreams, my clients re-learn how to recognize intuitive moments in their daily lives, and to again trust the accuracy of those intuitions. Perhaps facilitated by the unconditional love they experience when in the presence of their guides, they also learn to better differentiate fear-based thoughts from intuition. As they increasingly recognize and value ordinary hunches in day-to-day living, they find they can more easily sidestep or defuse situations that previously would have felt stressful. Life becomes more playful, more intriguing, as "coincidences" are increasingly understood as more literally linked to their thoughts, feelings, and intentions.

As you read their stories, I hope their messages will have a similar effect for you. Pay attention to places in the book where something that you read seems to strike a resonant chord in you. Resist the temptation to just keep reading. Pause for a moment and sit with your feelings. Instead of trying to analyze their source, imagine giving yourself permission to turn a dial that allows you to experience these feelings even more intensely. Play with the possibility that it was no coincidence that you had the reaction you did to what you had just read. Invite your intuitive sense to elaborate on the message being conveyed by what you are feeling.

Most people who experience an NDE encounter some form of non-physical being or guide. As will be evident throughout the book, I personally believe that every person has one or more such guides who are available during life and not just after physical death. Whatever your beliefs about the form and function of guides, you can use unexpected moments of intense feelings as a kind of "affect bridge" to help you and your guide(s) communicate better with each other. Similar to leaving a message on a close friend's cell phone without focusing on how the message actually gets there, imagine sending a message to your guide that explicitly gives him or her permission to use this window of opportunity to offer you guidance, suggestions, or support.

Chapter 2
Near-Death Experiences: A Brief Review

Since at least the mid-1970s, a number of researchers have described a consistent cluster of experiences that people report having had during a near-death experience. These life-changing experiences most often occur following a heart attack or other traumatic event during which the person's vital signs stop, and end when the person is resuscitated. More recently, researchers have also reported on "shared" near-death experiences in which someone else who is present has the same, concurrent experience as the "dead" person —but without the life-threatening physical component.

Not every person experiences every aspect of this cluster during a near-death experience. Taken collectively, though, the interview data remains strikingly consistent. Ring (1985) and Sabom (1982) have summarized similar sets of core transcendental experiences. Combining the two results in the following common core characteristics:

1. A subjective sense of being dead.

The person has the clear awareness that his/her physical body was dead.

2. Feelings of peace, painlessness, pleasantness, etc. (core affective cluster).

In sharp contrast to the physical sensations just a few seconds before (such as the crushing chest pain associated with a heart attack), the person reports a sudden, complete sense of peace and the total absence of pain or any other type of physical or emotional discomfort.

3. A sense of bodily separation.

The person becomes aware of moving out of the body, typically floating a few feet above it. There have been many, many reported cases of the person later describing quite accurately what was going on in the vicinity of the body; for example, words spoken by medical personnel, or actions taken by other people to resuscitate the body.

4. A sense of entering the dark region.

If the experience lasts long enough, the person has a sense of leaving the area where the body is and entering a dark region or tunnel.

5. Encountering a presence/hearing a voice.

At some point in the process, many report becoming aware of a presence, or of hearing one or more voices. Sometimes this is a previously deceased loved one. Sometimes the being is described in religious or angelic terms. The emotional tone of the meeting is one of feeling exquisitely safe.

6. Taking stock of one's life.

Usually in the presence of this being, the person begins a full review of his/her life. This process is reported as taking place in a manner that is totally non-judgmental. People report a sense that there is no possible way of trying to hide unflattering information or of altering the truth of events that took place during their lives. In the environment, absent of any hint of being scolded or chided, the person is able to experience this life review in such a way that much is learned.

7. Seeing, or being enveloped in, light.

If the experience lasts long enough, most report seeing, or being surrounded by, an incredible white light. Many report a sense of being loved with an intensity that is seldom, if ever, known during their lifetimes. The small percentage of people who report having had an unpleasant NDE usually do not make it this far. One theory is that the physical body is successfully resuscitated sooner, probably while the person was still in the dark void. Thus, the person's logical belief is that there is nothing after physical death except this void.

8. Seeing beautiful colors.

Some report also seeing colors unlike any on Earth. Often, objects have a glow or shimmering quality to them.

9. Entering into the Light.

Following the life review, some report a sense of moving into the Light as if beginning to travel towards its source. In conjunction with the next aspect of some NDEs, a few people report reaching a threshold beyond which they are told they are not allowed to go. At this junction, some are given a choice about whether they will return to their bodies. Others are told that it is not yet their time and they must go back.

10. Encountering visible "spirits".

Those who had not already seen a being/guide/angel or loved one during the NDE sometimes see one after they enter the Light. This figure sometimes serves as an escort.

11. A return to the physical body.

Obviously, the only NDEs that we know of involve people who were successfully resuscitated. Those who choose to come back often report that their reason for returning was because they wanted to continue in an important relationship such as with a parent or spouse, or they wanted to complete an unfinished project of significance. For many who were told they had to come back, the knowledge that they would be returning from this exquisitely peaceful place to a body that had been, moments before, in great physical pain, was news that was not well received!

When my therapy clients experience the death of the fictional person they were in a waking dream, they report very similar experiences to those of a true NDE. These occur independent of both the person's religious background and prior knowledge of NDE phenomena. Again, not all of the phenomena are experienced by each client, but the pattern includes the following:

1. Clients report a sense of floating out of the body (OBE) of the dream character at the moment of death. They typically report looking down at the body.

2. Clients report an intense calm, tranquility, and/or peacefulness.

While the intent of waking dreams is not to deal directly with client's beliefs about death and dying, such experiences seem to have an implicit impact on those beliefs.

3. Clients engage in a life-review experience in which they survey their dream life much as described in the NDE literature.

Unlike true NDEs, however, after retracing his or her life in trance, the client can return to a critical life moment in the waking dream and substitute a different action based on the insight gained from the life-review experience. Following the experience of living out the revised decision, the dream character dies a second time and conducts a second life review. This allows a more complete comparison of the consequences associated with each alternative, with full emotional involvement.

4. For many clients, if not most, there is a sense of the presence of a guide or angel or significant "other" person who facilitates the life review and helps provide important insights or perspectives.

This non-judgmental interpersonal hypnotic experience is quite a contrast for the client who has had a long history of being criticized both by others and by his or her own overly rigid conscience. The willingness to be introspective is enhanced by the complete absence of any judgmental tone to the experience. I find that clients who are normally defensive when not in trance show no evidence of being defensive during this part of the waking dream.

5. Some clients report profound experiences of insight, unconditional love, or forgiveness by themselves and/or by the ones they define as guides or angels or God.

I am careful to let clients define these experiences for themselves, and avoid superimposing my own beliefs, labels, or interpretations. Some clients describe this as experiencing a kind of total vulnerability matched with total safety and acceptance. Clients often have trouble putting the experience into words, but their joyful facial expressions convey much of the intensity of what they are feeling! The client's religious background appears to be largely unrelated to the form and content of these experiences.

6. The classic NDE experience ends with the person returning to his or her physical body and subsequently regaining consciousness.

By contrast, in waking dreams, the dream character who has died does not return to his/her physical body and resume living. Instead, clients often describe a sense of watching the character go off into the Light, often accompanied by a loved one or some type of spiritual being.

In the next chapter, we'll explore in more detail how these characteristics of an NDE present in a typical waking dream.

Chapter 3
A Typical Waking Dream

Initiating a waking dream in therapy is straightforward. The experience is very much like having a daydream. While most clients choose to lie down on the couch and close their eyes, some remain in a seated position with their eyes open. I have even experienced some of my own waking dreams while pacing back and forth in a room. Just like when we daydream, it is easier to have a waking dream when the person is relaxed physically and emotionally. One simple way I help my clients do this is to have them remember a time when they were feeling relaxed in this way. For some, this means walking in a grassy meadow. For others, it may involve sitting along a river bank. Some choose a walk along a forest path with the sun shining through the trees.

I frequently use the following teaching exercise with my clients. If you want, try this experience for yourself:

> Remember a classroom from your years in elementary school. It doesn't matter which one you choose or even if it is from a later time period. Imagine yourself in the classroom and notice the color of the chalkboard. Now look at the wall above the chalkboard and notice what you see there. Most people report seeing cards with the letters of the alphabet. If that happens to be what you see, notice the color of the cards and the color of the letters. Now walk up to the chalkboard and find a piece of chalk that is a good length. What color did you choose? Notice if you can feel the chalky texture when you pick it up. Then draw or write something on the board. When you're done, put the chalk back on the chalk tray. Did you notice the sound of the chalk as you wrote or when you put it back down? Finally, look for an eraser. Notice if there is already chalk dust on it or if it is clean. Erase what you wrote or drew on the board. Is it completely gone or is there a faint image left?

If you did the exercise yourself, it is likely that the image you had of the classroom was based on a real memory. At the point where I ask the client to write on the board, the experience most likely becomes purely fictional. A few people retrieve a memory of a time when they wrote something on the board during class, but for most, this part of the experience is fictional. However, nothing in the quality of the imagery changes when the content moves from the real memory to one which is fictional. The sights, sounds, and feelings seem very similar if not identical. This is why I'm very careful in how I use hypnosis/imagery. For the purpose of waking dreams, I arbitrarily define the content as fictional. This is easy to do since the person is *always* someone else in the dream. If you did the exercise yourself, notice how tall you were when you walked up to the chalkboard in your mind. Most people report that they were the height of a child, not their adult height, even though I said nothing specific about *being* younger in the exercise. Waking dreams take advantage of the mind's ability to imagine in a multi-sensory, even multi-age way.

After I help clients move into a relaxed trance state, I ask them to imagine being in a movie or story whose main character's life will contain experiences that they will find meaningful and relevant. For example, I may say, "As you continue to relax and go even more deeply within, you might find yourself beginning to imagine being someone in a movie; a person whose story will contain experiences that will be *timely, useful, and constructive* for you in your own life." While I could certainly offer more specific suggestions, I like to keep the risks of biasing or confounding the process to a minimum by being as non-specific as possible. In this way, whatever imagery emerges for the client has the best chance of being generated independent of any beliefs I may have about the nature or origin of the client's issues. There are many ways to phrase this opening suggestion. One way is to ask the client's unconscious or higher self "to generate a story, perhaps from another time and place, in which the events will provide you with greater understanding of (the current concern) that will be constructive, timely, and useful in helping you to resolve it".

For several years, one of my favorite ways of helping a client initiate a waking dream has been to use an extension of the "Hallway of Doors" hypnotic technique that I call "The Atrium". A sample induction follows.

20

Sample induction for The Atrium:

Induction	Discussion
As you let your eyes close and continue to relax even more, imagine you are standing in a hallway with many closed doors. As you look down the hallway, the door nearest you is number 43. Behind that door are all of the memories of everything that has happened in this year of your life. Beyond that, as you look farther down the hallway, there is a door for every year in your life so far.	Assume the client is currently 43 years old.

It is my personal preference to actively discourage clients from using this tool to explore their future. Imagine, for example, a client who only sees two additional doors and concludes that she will die at age 45. |
| Behind you, the hallway continues, perhaps around a corner. The doors in that part of the hallway have not yet been installed to hold all of the memories for each of the years that await you in this life. | The "Hallway of Doors" is typically used to explore antecedents of current problems. Using trance-deepening language, the client is invited to walk along the hallway until she reaches the door "behind which can be found the origin of the problem", or "where you can find memories that relate to the origin of the problem". |
| As you walk, at your own pace, past each of the doors moving farther down the hallway, you can allow your mind to go deeper and deepr within, becoming even more relaxed and comfortable. As you continue, you can make a mental note of any thoughts | This reduces the risk of an unexpected abreaction in cases where a client has memories that are still painful. This is particularly important if the client's childhood history includes correlates that are often found in cases where significant abuse occurred. |

or feelings that occur as you pass by each of the doors. The memories from those years will stay safely secure behind the closed doors. If you'd like, you can let me know how far down the hallway you have already gone, noticing the number on the door nearest you.	
When you reach the end of the hallway, it opens into an atrium. This is a private place designed just for you. For some, the atrium has beautiful white light streaming in from windows located high above. For others, it is smaller and more cozy. Your atrium may have pathways lined with plants or flowers. There may be a small pond or even a fountain or waterfall. When you're ready, take a moment, and describe what you're noticing.	The imagery is designed to be very safe. I tell clients that even I am not allowed to go there. The intent of these permissively worded suggestions is to further convey the sense that being in the atrium is equated with feeling very peaceful, calm, etc. A few clients describe an outdoor setting for their atrium.
As you look around the edges of the atrium, you may notice other hallways, similar to the one that brought you here. Like hallways in a large movie theater, each of these other hallways can serve as the entry point for you into a waking dream. When you're ready, you can invite your higher self to guide you towards a hallway that is just right for today. As you	I prefer the term "higher self" to that of the "unconscious". The latter term is often associated with negative

move into the hallway, your mind can carry you effortlessly, at the speed of thought, across time and space to the opening scene of the dream.

During the dream, if something unpleasant occurs, you can, if you want, return to the atrium at the speed of thought, or you can simply let your eyes open. If you are willing, though, stay with the experience and tell me what is happening so that I may help you with it.

When you are ready, let me know what you've been noticing.

connotations. In practice, I use whatever term the client is most comfortable using.

Just twice, I've had a client whose initial foray into the atrium felt threatening. It is critical to address this, much as one would do with dream interpretation, exploring the symbolic meaning of the threat.

Sometimes a client will say, "I just see black," or, "I don't see anything." When this occurs, I find the following usually works well:

First, I assess if it is "black/dark" in all directions. If the client has made such an observation, it usually is.

Then I ask, "Would you like a flashlight or a lantern to help you see more clearly?" Most clients choose a flashlight. The client will typically respond with a comment like, "Oh, there's a door in front of me."

If this is insufficient, I shift to a different sensory modality. For example, tactile questions:
- "Notice if your feet are touching anything."

	• "If you reach out with your hand, notice what you feel." One client responded, "I feel a cold, slightly damp stone wall." I had her feel her way along the wall until she found a way out of the dark space.
	Auditory questions:
	• "Are you aware of any sound?"
	• "If you speak, does your voice echo?"
	Kinesthetic questions:
	• "Notice the air temperature in this dark space."
	• "Are you abel to move?"
	Cognitive questions:
	• "Imagine sending a thought to the darkness. Ask the darkness what function it is attempting to serve for you."
	The response often involves a theme of protection. As in the story below involving the tiger, I have the client explore the theme with the reified darkness as if using mental telepathy.

In practice, the dream is almost always experienced in the first person rather than the third person, so the dream is richly emotional and not just a cognitive experience. In fact, when the client does experience the dream in the third person as an observer, it seems to serve a protective function that allows the person some emotional distance from the content of the dream. I do not use waking dreams to access real memories from childhood. Indeed, when a history of childhood trauma is suspected, skilled therapists know that any use of hypnosis must be done with considerable caution.

For some, the waking dream begins with an experience of being a child. For others, the person is already an adult. The entry point is not critical, other than that I suggest letting it begin at a point where things are calm. It's no fun to have an opening scene that seems like something out of a war movie. On the rare occasions when this happens, I suggest the client "fast forward" or "rewind" the experience to a point where things are more settled.

Because the dream content is arbitrarily defined as fictional, it is even workable to have the client intentionally make up an initial scene. For example, one client, Eric, kept rejecting images he was having because he thought he was consciously making them up, and thought they should somehow feel different if his unconscious was generating them. I suggested he simply make up a scene. Eric immediately saw himself—as a different person, Randall—approaching a fork on a dirt road at which stood a large, dead tree. As he studied the image, he had a sense the area had suffered a severe drought for several years. Turning down the left fork, Randall came to an abandoned house, which triggered profound sadness. As the waking dream continued, its theme and mood had clear parallels to the long-standing emotional drought in the client's marriage and the "fork in the road" he had come to in his life. Eric's dream is presented in full in Chapter 6.

Another client, Amanda, had a waking dream that began with a rather frightening scene. She experienced herself being at the bottom of a ravine. She became quite scared to see a large tiger at the top of the ravine looking down at her. I reminded her she could leave the dream if she wanted, but asked her if she would imagine sending a thought to the tiger that she was scared. When she did, I watched a puzzled look come over her face. "What happened?" I asked. She said, "The tiger sent back a thought that it is scared of *me!*" I invited her to dialogue mentally with the tiger about this (since they could obviously exchange thoughts without actually speaking in the dream) and see how they might resolve this in a manner that was agreeable to both. She lay silent for a moment or two and then announced calmly, "I'm riding on his back now. We're going to travel together." We can certainly speculate about the symbolism of the tiger in her dream. I did not comment at the time as it seemed unnecessary—she resolved the fear herself. One possibility is that her apprehension about what she might learn about herself through the vehicle of waking dreams presented in the form of the tiger. Another possibility is that the tiger represented the masculine side of her persona. Whatever the true meaning, when she confronted her fear in this symbolic way, she found a way to reframe the adrenalin rush from anxiety and apprehension to curiosity and courage.

Most waking dreams follow a chronological progression over the life of the main character. Sometimes events are experienced out of sequence. Some clients will describe considerable contextual details regarding the person's life. Others offer only minimal details like a theater stage with very few props. Sometimes the dreams include the names of people, cities, or even specific years. If asked about such information, however, the client typically reports that the details are unimportant.

Most people have an easy time seeing things in their mind's eye. Some who have a much harder time with visual images are able to hear sounds. Still others have strong kinesthetic/feeling experiences. As noted above, if a client is having trouble generating visual imagery, I shift to asking about sounds or feelings, or I may ask questions aimed at providing more context:

> "You might notice what you are wearing, if anything, on your feet."
> "What time of day or night does it seem to be?"
> "Do you have a sense of being indoors or outside?"
> "Notice if you sense the presence of another person."
> "Do you hear any sounds?"

If the client encounters emotionally intense content, there are a variety of ways of handling it. One strategy is the "screening room" technique. I have clients imagine they are sitting in a small theater or screening room with me. In their mind, they hold a remote control device like that used for VCRs that they can use to control the dream in a variety of ways. They can fast forward over a scary scene in the dream, or pause the action while I help them relax. Similarly, they can mute the sound in the dream, analogous to turning down the volume during the scary part of a movie so that the sound effects are not heard. In the screening room, emotional intensity is automatically toned down by shifting to a third-person perspective where the client is watching the movie on the screen rather than being in the movie in the first person. As an alternative, I may have the client simply shift to a third-person vantage point within the dream and move to a safe distance to observe what is happening. For example, "If you'd like, step back and watch what is happening, *now*, from a safe vantage point."

Many clients pace the life of the dream character in a way that I am able to remain mostly silent, recording what they tell me about the experience. If I sense the momentum is slowing, I will suggest something like, "And when you are ready, you can let the scene move to the next important event which will be useful for you to see." In practice, once the client has become the dream character, I refer to the dream character as "you" rather than "he" or "she". It is easier for the client to stay in character in the dream experience this way. For example, "You can let yourself notice whether there is anything else about what is happening now that it is important for you to understand in a conscious way."

When the life of the person in the dream seems to be nearing its end, I may suggest, "If it is okay, I'd like to ask you to move ahead in time to the end of your life [as the dream character]." If the client is experiencing the dream from a third-person perspective, I will honor that by changing the language. For example, if the dream character is identified as Claire, I may suggest, "You can move ahead in time to the end of Claire's life." For many, this is sufficient to prompt a scene just prior to the person's death. If not, I may offer suggestions aimed at helping the client set the stage. "You might notice the circumstances ... where you are ... whether anyone else is present ... what is happening *now*." In practice, I never suggest the specifics of how the person in the dream dies. When invited to explore the final part of the life of the person in the dream, most clients spontaneously include the death of the person. I *rarely* need to intervene as the person dies. Clients rarely report emotional distress of such intensity that they are reluctant to let the process continue. For the rare client who seems to be in some distress, I invite him or her to view what is happening "from a safe distance", or I might suggest, "You can let yourself safely float up above this scene *now* and notice how it ends." A reaction of some distress is more likely to occur if the death in the dream was violent or the result of an accident such as a drowning. In such situations, I use standard hypnotic techniques for helping tone down the emotional intensity of the experience. For example, I may remind the person, "You can observe what is happening to Claire knowing that you are safe here in my office and need not experience in *your* physical body any discomfort that is happening to Claire's body." Using the screening room notion of a remote control device, I may suggest, "You can fast forward over this part to notice the outcome." I find that suggestions such as this quickly serve to abate any acute anxiety symptoms. Following the death, with very rare exceptions, there is an immediate shift to a sense of complete peacefulness and calm. Knowing that, it is much easier for the client to go back and review the final moments when the death was a traumatic one.

At the moment in the dream when death occurs, most clients report a significant shift in how they feel. Again, this is particularly true if the death was secondary to some kind of accident or other trauma. Regardless of the circumstances leading to the death, most spontaneously float out of the body of the dream character. Independent of the nature of the death, they report feeling very calm, tranquil, and at peace. Because this part of the experience is so consistently associated with the absence of any judgmental tone or attitude, it creates an emotionally safe environment within which the client may review and self-critique the dream content. As is the norm in the NDE literature, clients seem very open and non-defensive as they explore the content and implications of the dream content from this out-of-body perspective.

I help them do this in a variety of ways:

1. They may review major decisions or conclusions, especially those made at the very end of the life.
2. They may notice pre-existing assumptions that were found to be invalid in the dream content.
3. Based on the life outcomes of the dream content, they may return to a critical decision point, enact a different choice, and live out the consequences of this new alternative as a way of experimenting with new solutions.

4. After the death of the person in the dream, I routinely propose a dialogue between the dream character and the client. The out-of-body person can be asked if he or she has any suggestions for the client regarding the client's own presenting issues based on the life experiences from the dream. The content of the suggestions that ensue are often predictable; however, the tone is usually quite different from that which typically characterizes internal self-talk. The tone of the person in the dream is described by clients in terms such as "gentle, non-judgmental, supportive, encouraging, forgiving". Sometimes the suggestions are thematic such as, "You're taking this issue much too seriously. Lighten up!" At other times the suggestions are very concrete and specific.

5. I often use a split-screen image to suggest that the client notice correlations between the dream life and his or her own life. Even without suggesting specific possibilities, many will report personality parallels between other people in the dream life and current relationships in the client's life. Just as Dorothy in *The Wizard of Oz* incorporated neighbors and family members in her dream experiences, clients often incorporate critical elements of their own relationships in waking dreams. These can be worked with in various ways to tease out faulty assumptions, to reframe aspects of the relationship, or to dialogue with the people involved in the dream about alternative solutions to the problem.

6. One fascinating outcome is when the client and the dream character agree on a signal (an operant conditioning cue) that the client will use in the future to remind himself or herself to use the new solution that was generated in this dialogue. When a particular symptom, such as acute anxiety, begins to emerge, the dream character or the guides respond with a cue. This cue alerts the client consciously to what is happening, and then triggers the opportunity to use a new, alternative response that the client has agreed will be more effective and emotionally calming.

7. If the presence of guides or angels is experienced, I focus on the emotional healing potential of a relationship, which has unconditional love as its foundation.

I make use of these guides as if they are co-therapists assisting me on behalf of my clients. I find the comfort, support, and suggestions that clients attribute to their guides to be consistently constructive and positive. Most present in human form in the client's imagery, though some present as animals or birds or fish. Most indicate that they have been with the client since birth. Occasionally, I encounter a guide who works with the client on a time-limited project. For example, while using hypnosis with a client to help her prepare for major surgery, I invited her to notice if her guides wanted to add any suggestions to the work we were doing that day. She reported that a new guide introduced himself as John. She said he told her that he would be with her just during the surgery and recovery period. When she was several weeks into her uneventful post-operative recovery period, she reported that John had visited with her once again to tell her that his work with her was now finished. In the months that followed, she had no further contact from him.

Another client who happens to have a Dissociative Identity Disorder (multiple personalities) called me one day in some distress. She told me she had just awoken from a nap and found that her room was full of people, some two dozen of them. I had worked with her for several years at that point, and knew she had no prior history of visual hallucinations. I asked her to notice if one of the people seemed to be a spokesperson for the group. She indicated there was. I suggested she ask, simply, why they were there. She did and reported that one of them told her, "Well, there are many of you so we figured that it would only be fair if there were enough of us to go around." Throughout her youth, she had consistently felt that she had to put her own needs second to those of other family members. Here, she understood without further discussion that this group was offering her—and every one of her alter personalities—a one-to-one relationship of support and guidance. In the years since that afternoon, whenever she has experienced significant emotional distress, she has been able to calm herself (and her other parts) in about thirty seconds by inviting this group of guides to be with her.

Another of my clients routinely worked with two guides, a male and a female, whom she experienced as standing on either side of her. They regularly nudged her to tell me something that she was reluctant to address. If they thought we were getting too far off on a tangent, they would tell her to tell me so—and she would. I firmly believe that her willingness to allow this kind of active involvement by her guides in her therapy was the result of the simple reality that their advice and manner of support has always been both on target and very loving.

When one of my clients first meets a guide such as the ones I have described above, I routinely pose a series of questions for the client to put to the guide(s). I invite the client to, "Notice the response you get to the question, and pay careful attention *to your own reaction* to that response." The critical message here is for the client to learn to trust his or her own intuition. If the client doesn't feel comfortable or trusting of the response from the guide, I pay careful attention to it. I make no assumption that when the client "sees" someone that this means I am dealing with a guide as opposed to there being some other explanation for what is happening. In practice, my clients report that the guide seems to know the rest of my question before I finish asking it, and that as the questions continue, the guide begins to grin in a knowing anticipation of the next question—to which the answer will also be an affirming, "Yes."

I begin by asking the client to inquire if the guide "is from the Light". While it is easy for someone to lie on a job application or personality test, it has been my experience that whomever or whatever these beings are, they do not lie. On very rare occasions when a client has asked this question, the person simply left. If the client has *any* reservation about the answer to this question, I follow with additional hypnotic techniques that usually resolve the uncertainty. Once the client is clear that the person/guide is "from the Light", I ask the client to confirm some assumptions that I have consistently found to be true. Assume the client's name is Jane.

> "Are you [the guide] available at any time, or do you keep office hours?"

I phrase it this way to call attention to the fact that guides are available at times when clients are often reluctant to call their therapist. I find guides are available at any hour of the day or night—weekends, holidays, and power failures included.

> "Do you promise that you will never try to 'make' Jane do anything; that you will only offer advice?"

31

I find that guides *never* "insist". They may remind, nudge, encourage, or prod, but they never insist or demand. They may comment about the consequences of procrastinating on an issue or the benefits of dealing with it, but they leave the decision up to the client. The only exception I have encountered involves situations in which the person has had an intuitive "knowing" that he or she had to react immediately, usually to avoid being injured.

> "Can Jane expect that if she asks a question, that you will answer it—if you are allowed to do so?"

I find that guides provide information in proportion to how often they are asked. They seldom intrude, but when asked for help they are quick to provide what they are able. They tend not to answer many specific questions about future-tense events. They will not tell someone what they "should" do. Their suggestions come as options, as possibilities that the person is free to use or not. One client wanted me to recommend some books for her to read. While I have my favorites that I thought might be useful, I suggested she go to a bookstore and ask her guides to point out some possibilities. She e-mailed me on her return from the store, somewhat stunned at the success of this new way of utilizing her guides whom she felt had steered her to two books that she found very relevant.

> "Is it true that you can be much more helpful to Jane if she specifically asks for your help?"

Good friends often wait to offer suggestions (only) when they are requested. I find guides are eager to help, but tend to be much more actively involved when we specifically ask them to do so. For example, having forgotten to take his pass key to get into his office building one Saturday, another client decided to do some shopping. He asked his guide, a hawk, about the idea of checking out one of two local exercise stores for some replacement equipment he was contemplating purchasing. He told me the hawk pointed him towards the second of the two stores. There he found the equipment he wanted—on sale—from a reputable manufacturer whose price was more than $1,000 lower than the brand he had planned to purchase. The salesman explained that the only difference was in the level of sophistication of the on-board computer.

Following a waking dream, I help the client return to a fully alert waking state. During trance, the body is usually very still and relaxed, so, on re-alerting, many report feeling as they would if they had just taken a nap or had a massage. This re-orienting is important to help insure that when clients drive out of the parking lot, their reaction times are back to normal. Hypnotic experiences often seem to move in non-linear time, and safely negotiating the traffic on the interstate near my office requires quick (linear) reaction times.

I avoid engaging in much discussion about the waking dream at the end of the session. I prefer to let the experience settle at its own pace over the rest of the day. Therefore, I usually reserve any analysis of its meaning until the next therapy session. Unlike the fleeting memories associated with nighttime dreams, clients remember most of the content of their waking dreams when they come out of trance. Just as they don't remember *every* detail of what was talked about during a regular therapy session, they don't remember every detail of a waking dream. To help reduce clients' concerns about possibly forgetting some important detail, I often audiotape waking dreams. Some clients like to listen to the tape from the session one or more times during the week. Like watching a good movie more than once, they find they gain additional ideas or insights in this manner. I also take detailed notes, so that when we do discuss the content of a waking dream, I can help remind the client of specific events or comments that were made.

Sometimes there isn't enough time in a single therapy session to finish the life's story of the dream character. On other occasions, the client and I both sense that there is more to be gleaned from returning to a particular part of the dream character's life and exploring it further. Just before ending the trance work, I may suggest that the client and the dream character agree to meet again to continue the story of the dream character's life. At a pragmatic level, they often choose a specific location in the imagery or a specific scene from the story, analogous to two friends agreeing to meet again at a coffee shop the following week to resume their conversation. If the client is going to do more work with the same waking dream, at the next session I will often summarize what took place in the previous session as a way to begin. Listening to the summary in this way is automatically trance inducing for most clients, facilitating an easy return to the imagery.

When clients discuss the meaning of a particular waking dream, it is usually obvious if they've made the connection between the theme(s) in the imagery and their personal lives. When a faulty assumption is uncovered, it quickly gives way to a new under-standing of the situation. At other times, a new solution emerges that the client begins to implement. Sometimes durable change occurs without any lengthy discussion of the dream's content. One woman came for therapy to deal with intense anger at her husband about some things he had done several years earlier in their mar-riage. She recognized that her anger was way out of proportion, but had been unable to let it go. I met with the couple for a few sessions to be sure I could find no other basis for her anger, and then sug-gested we utilize hypnosis. Her husband showed up in two of her waking dreams. In one, both she and her husband had been (male) warriors on opposing sides in a battle. The woman's dream charac-ter had been killed by the other warrior. The other waking dream involved a second variation on this theme. Following these two ses-sions, her anger at her husband disappeared. At follow up several months later, her husband concurred with her opinion that the anger had durably dissipated.

One direct consequence of these kinds of experiences is that my clients report a shift in how they understand the "coincidences" that occur in their lives. While it is not my intent to "prove" that most coincidences can have other explanations, I find that my clients evolve a different attitude about life's unexpected quirks. They come to react to them as unexpected possibilities, cleverly disguised in many different ways, which they would have previ-ously labeled as annoying or inconvenient. As I was editing this very paragraph one day, a client "misremembered" the time for a scheduled phone consult and called three hours early. During the time that remained, I had intended to make a critical, difficult call to someone on her behalf, which we had been planning for quite awhile. The client and I reconfirmed the later phone time and started to say goodbye. Before we hung up, she took a moment to tell me about a conversation she had had the night before that eliminated the need for me to make the call. We both chuckled at the suspicion that our respective guides had a hand in the "coincidences" involved in the timing of her call, as she had not known that I would be making my call just before we were scheduled to talk. Whether or not guides played a role in this particular situation, my clients and I find life is much more intriguing when we approach the unexpected with an attitude of curiosity and anticipation.

In the following chapters, we'll explore a variety of ways in which the different experiences that clients have manifest in waking dreams. Each client has given his or her permission to use the transcript of the waking dream. While names and identifying information have been changed to protect confidentiality, very little editing has been done of the actual dream content.

Chapter 4
"Now Go Paint the Rest of Your Life"

Dorothy

A traumatic event sometimes has the effect of putting life on hold for an extended period of time. Trauma can trigger grief because of a tangible loss or because of the shattering of a belief. A number of years ago, Elisabeth Kübler-Ross helped define six stages of grieving. She noted that the stages do not move sequentially, but more like waves, where at any given moment the next wave may land at a different place on the shore. The six components: denial, anger, bargaining, depression/sadness, acceptance/resignation, and growth occur over time naturally and in a manner that is idiosyncratic to the person and the event. If a person gets stuck in a particular aspect of the grieving, it can be like driving a car with the parking brake not fully released: it puts a drag on the ability to move forward with life.

One client, Dorothy, had had just such a traumatic event. She was referred to me by her neurologist because of some lingering symptoms secondary to a car accident that had occurred some 18 months before. She had been a passenger in a car that was hit from behind. The impact pushed the car into the car ahead of her. She had developed classic symptoms of post traumatic stress disorder (PTSD). For at least a year following the accident, she was unable to drive because of dizziness that would occur at unpredictable times. She had other unpleasant neurological symptoms, such as periods of confusion and tiring easily. The accident had brought most of her independence to a sudden halt. Her way of life, as she had known it, had come to an abrupt end.

Over a period of several months, Dorothy had a series of waking dreams that incorporated symbolic aspects of how the accident had impacted her life. The first several of these each included a sudden death. At the end of a long, simple life in one dream, the man (Harry) died suddenly of a massive heart attack. Greeted by relatives who had died before him, he was aware of both wanting to be with them and of being anxious to go back to another existence. At a symbolic level, his wish could be understood as a metaphor for Dorothy's wish to be able to go back to the way things were and have another chance at life.

In Dorothy's second waking dream as a young widow (Anne) during World War II, she was struck and killed by a car while crossing a street as a pedestrian. As she floated above the body, I asked Dorothy to notice Anne's final thoughts. Speaking about Anne in the third person, Dorothy told me:

> She's [*Anne*] confused. She didn't know, didn't really know what happened and why it happened so quickly. She knows she was hit by a car, but doesn't accept that her life is over. It was too sudden.

This matched Dorothy's own experience following her car accident. Prior to the accident, she had led an independent life as a single woman running her own small business, a business that required considerable time spent in the car. Suddenly, she had found herself totally dependent on others for such simple things as getting to a grocery store. She had found it quite difficult to accept such basic help from other people. In the waking dream, Dorothy first helped Anne resolve her confusion and disbelief. Then she helped Anne reunite in the Light with her husband. In exchange, Anne offered to return the favor:

> She wants to help me. She sees my cloudiness, my confusion. She doesn't think she can clear it all by herself. She's touching my head, giving peace and happiness. She keeps embracing me, telling me to be strong, to keep working at it ... She wants to keep helping me. I see her saying she'll be with me, watching. She's extending her hands, touching my head to try to make things better. I feel calmer when she touches me. Almost like we've gone from being friends and companions to her watching for me, her taking care of me. ["*Is that okay with you?*" *I asked.*] Yes. I trust her.

At this point, I helped Dorothy create an operant conditioning cue as described in Chapter 3. In its basic form, if A happens, it will trigger B to happen. In this case, I helped her anchor Anne's calming touch (B) as a response to future feelings of cognitive cloudiness (A). Then I built on this idea of Anne serving as a resource by inviting her to notice if there were others who could help:

> **Therapist:** Then in the future if you are feeling some of that cloudiness, can she come and touch your head to restore that sense of calm and peacefulness?
>
> **Client:** Yes. I was there for her to help her; she'll do what she can to help me. Now our roles are reversed. She'll help me find a way back as much as she can.
>
> **Therapist:** As you helped her to find her husband, can she bring others to you who may also help?
>
> **Client:** Yes. There is an aura of purple around her helping her. I don't see anyone behind her but I feel tremendous help through her for me. I catch glimpses of my father [*who had died a decade earlier*] now and then; the rest is just an energy or aura around her. It's very big. It's all very positive, very loving, very warm. They want to do all they can ... I feel she and everyone with her will really be there for me. They won't be able to do it all. She's telling me she won't do everything, but will always be there whenever I need her. They'll be there to give me strength, guidance, the capacity to go forward.

The power of this largely invisible group is similar to the client who awoke from a dream one afternoon to find a room full of people who came to provide support. For Dorothy and the other client, I think the experience conveys two implicit messages: First, whatever the client's problem, the group is big enough to handle it. Second, the emotional heaviness of the problem won't be a burden to the group the way it could be for a single caregiver.

As the images drew to a close, Dorothy commented:

> I don't see the purple any more. It's just all lighter. There is warmth around her [*Anne*] that comes into me through her hands.

A few months later, Dorothy experienced an application of another operant conditioning cue I had created during her hypnosis work. This one occurred when she was driving home one evening after dark. Three weeks earlier, we had done some hypnosis work recalling a multi-state car trip she had driven solo during her early twenties. She had begun that trip with some doubts about her ability to complete it. I had helped her anchor her emerging confidence with a visual image that was to re-emerge on this nighttime drive home from another part of the state. She noted that she had begun to have problems with the oncoming headlights and the white lines in the road beginning to visually cross. She reported a sudden shift in experience as she heard my voice (from the earlier session) telling her that the center line was her anchor and the stars were her guide. She reported that she immediately relaxed and did much better the rest of the drive home.

Like watching a good movie several times and noticing things that were overlooked before, Dorothy returned to the theme of sudden loss in her next waking dream. In this one, she was again a man (George) who had married and raised two children. In his later years, he suffered a stroke, which left him unable to speak for the few days before he died. She noted that, "He didn't feel robbed because his life ended early. He's just sorry he couldn't talk with his family at the end." That led into a dialogue between Dorothy and George in which he cautioned her:

> He's telling me to not let that happen to me. To always express my emotions and feelings every day, *because you don't know if you'll have a next time to talk with people* ... [*A few years after this session, George's advice came to seem prophetic, as you will see at the end of this chapter.*] Again, he expresses sorrow at not being able to express himself at the end. He tells me to really work at what I'm going through now so that I don't have to go through these limitations.

Following up on the neurological implications of a stroke in her dream symbolism, I asked Dorothy to scan her body for parallels. She commented:

> That's what he's telling me. This [*the stroke*] happened to him, not to me. It's all his, not mine. He's telling me to put all those thoughts and confusions behind me.

> I see George and Anne now, both there to help me. What happened to them is not to be reflected in me ... I feel like they're telling me there are other lives. They are happy I've recognized in my own experience the value of what's important and what isn't—the

people we love and not possessions, not work. An understanding of the value of life. They're saying it will enrich my relationships with family and friends. This deepens them even more than before. I've learned to give up fear by being willing to ask for help. It's sharing of help whenever anyone needs support. They say I need to get more rest so my brain can heal even more.

At the end of that session, she commented again how difficult it had previously been for her to accept help. The clear message she heard from Anne and George went in at both the literal and metaphorical level: "It's okay (to ask for help). We're happy to do it. You've done it for us." For several years after that waking dream, she confirmed that it had become easier both to ask for help and to accept it when offered.

Three months after her waking dream as Anne, Dorothy returned for a second look at Anne's life. As Anne, she focused on the time period between her husband's death and her own death. We followed that with a "what if" sequence in the dream. For Dorothy, this meant allowing herself to play out in the dream the "what if" had Anne not been killed in the accident. Because, by definition, the "what if" is rarely possible in real life, sometimes a person can get stuck fantasizing about it, often in the form of, "If only ..."

Client: I feel like she [*Anne*] was really kind of lost after he [*Anne's husband*] died. Not knowing what to do with her time or what direction to take. Not long after she learned of his death, she was still making plans to go back home; to go back to her family for the healing process from his death. She'd never really worked because they had married and she did volunteer work there. But I feel she was a very independent person. She would have made it, pulled life together. She was going back home to regroup.

Therapist: Consider playing out Anne's life in a "what if" had she not died.

Client: [*Pause.*] I see her working with children in an orphanage or school or charity hospital because the children affected her so deeply. She would have lived at home with her family. She would have married again. I really do see she would have taught young children. She was involved beyond just being a teacher. I think she would have had a happy life.

41

Therapist: Then when you're ready, moving to the end of her life, into the Light, pausing to reflect on these choices.

Client: I see she did have a happy life with children of her own and another loving husband. I see how different one moment can make in a life. Like, one turn in the road, how different one path would be as opposed to the other.

Therapist: Notice any parallels between Anne's life and your own situation now of a different path. You might ask Anne for suggestions she may have.

Client: I feel she's touching me again. She's saying she didn't have the choice. I'm grateful I did; I still have my life. It can still be good. This can be dealt with. Maybe it will go away; it will be dealt with. She's saying, "Enjoy the gift of life." [*Pause.*] She's leaving me now. I feel better though. She's not here with me but is looking down. She'll be with me when I need her. I feel better just having been with her.

Therapist: If it's important, confirm that you can call on her.

Client: Yes, she'll always be near.

This dream sequence helped punctuate a theme that was to re-emerge in other dreams: this accident didn't kill you. You still have the option to go forward with your life. Similar to Anne's "what if" scenario, Dorothy had enacted her own "what if" change of direction since starting therapy. She had sold her business and joined with several others in starting up a new business that did not require her to be out on the road.

In the dream sequence presented below, Dorothy and the woman in the dream, Claire, have a lovely dialogue about this notion of moving forward. The catalyst for the dream was to explore hypnotically some ways to strengthen her visual processing skills since certain tasks continued to be difficult for her since the car accident.

Therapist: As I was rereading some of my notes this morning, I remembered that the first time we used hypnosis we began with what for you was an image of your home as a child, and that soft green color that embodied that wonderful sense of safety and comfort and, of course, at later times, we have used the beach imagery. So I invite you to pick one of those—or a different image—as a place to once again let the body remember that wonderful sense of comfort and relaxation, and to call on the remembrance of those we have met on other journeys, in other stories, whether Anne or George or your dad or all of those and more, as we look today for a story from another time and place where the kinds of things that you were so good at serve as a reference point, a kind of prototype, that we can draw on today as a means of rebuilding (neurological) pathways for anything which may still have been impacted from the accident. And so, as we do, to move easily across time and space surrounded by a beautiful beam of light, traveling safely at the speed of thought and touching down into a place and time where the story that emerges … the life of one who is central to the story, contains those elements that are right on target with the goals of today's session.

Client: I see myself just being drawn up and out of my room when I was a teenager, last living at home, up into the air and crossing a body of water … again, it feels like going back to the British Isles. I see the surf crashing against rocks and the shore. Again, I feel myself walking on a hilltop away from the shoreline. It's a sunny day. It's not a lush landscape, there are just a few trees here and there … tall grass blowing in the breeze. Almost feels like I'm a child. I go there with my father … just dancing around as he's walking. We're going back home. It's just a happy day. I see myself just laughing and playing around as he's walking us back. I see a girl in a long dress … eight years old keeps coming to mind.

Therapist: And, as always, you can move forward or backward in time so that you can become familiar with each point that would be useful or significant.

Client: I was just seeing myself back at our home, inside the home. We're cooking dinner, other children around. Now it feels like I'm a teenager in that same home. But still there are other children, other brothers and sisters. It's like we're talking about me going away to school somewhere. It feels like London and I'll be staying with relatives. I see horse-drawn carriages in the streets, cobblestone streets. It's like it would be unusual for me to go to school, but because I really want it so much, the family has made special arrangements. Now I can see myself walking in the streets with long dresses, a long coat, some kind of a hat or bonnet tied around my neck, carrying a large portfolio kind of thing under my arm.

Therapist: And how have your studies been going?

43

Client: I'm very happy. I see a drawing class. I see myself taking off the bonnet, spreading out my pencils, charcoals. There are mostly men in the class, just a few girls. Looks like we've gone through all kind of different lessons with objects and dimensions and landscapes and nudes. Now it's more still life … seeing the shading. I'm really happy. There's a group of students with several people and we're all very close and help each other.

I see one young man I'm getting especially close with. Now it seems we're married and we're in the south of France, just on those cliffs together drawing. Feels like watercolors. Yes, I like watercolors and he likes working with oils. I like the softness of the watercolors.

Therapist: Does this also serve as a way that the two of you can enjoy doing something that on the one hand is the same and yet not really competing with each other because the medium is different?

Client: Yes, I guess it could be that way. Sounds right in that we like feeding and interacting with each other with the different mediums we're interested in, critiquing each other's work. But we are never upset with the suggestions of the other. I see it as happy discussions. He just called my name. It's Claire.

Therapist: And just for fun, at some point you might hear yourself or someone else saying his name.

Client: Yes, I was saying "Joseph" as if I use his full name when I'm teasing him. We have a small bungalow. We do a lot of our work there but we like going out and doing landscapes. I see one room in the bungalow that's really bright, with lots of windows, and it's where we have the easels set up.

Therapist: I don't know if it matters whether the painting that the two of you do is how you support yourselves or whether there is some other way that the two of you derive the funds necessary to take care of the cost of living.

Client: I see us painting all the time. We're comfortable in our living, not wealthy, but have plenty of money to live a nice life. I see myself pregnant now, but still painting. I see how funny it looks to be pregnant in those big, long dresses! They are very comfortable dresses for being at home and working. I have a daughter. We're all so happy.

Therapist: What name did the two of you choose?

Client: Beth … Elizabeth, but we call her Beth. We're still doing our painting together. She's a toddler now, just running around with us. We enjoy our days of going out to the fields whether it's to paint the landscapes, or the sea, or the fields of flowers … and the fact that we can all be together while we're doing this. I see a little gallery where our work is. We're taking in some new paintings. It's just a small, little shop in the village … white walls, cobble streets again.

Therapist: Is this down in France or back in England or somewhere else?

Client: No, we're still in France. Still feels like the south of France. We are near the ocean—not the ocean, the Mediterranean.

Therapist: Does that mean that the two of you have learned somewhere along the way to be conversant in French?

Client: Yes, it's our home now.

Therapist: Out of curiosity, check back and notice when you first began learning French and what age.

Client: It feels like when I met Joseph at school. He was from France. That's why we went back there.

Therapist: Learning a foreign language as an adult is very different than being bi-lingual during early childhood. If it would be important or useful, you might replay some of what that experience was like as the interest and motivation to acquire a second language—a second way of communicating with words—came to be, and how you learned to develop all that is associated linguistically with being able to store and retrieve information from two languages, stored in one place.

Client: I knew just a little French before meeting Joseph and he was very fluent in English because he had planned to go to the school in London, so he had learned English early. Then as we became serious, that's when he began teaching me French. He teases me about my accent. I feel I was a very bright person so that learning it was not that difficult and the fact that once we were engaged, we mostly … he would speak mostly French with me, so it would be an everyday thing … exposure to it.

I see myself still thinking in English but having to convert it to the French. I'm happy that Beth will grow up with both languages. We speak mostly French, predominately since we're living there. But I do want her to know English and as she's a little older, I start teaching her. I didn't want to confuse her so much when she was very young, learning to talk.

Therapist: And as you've done each time that we visit the life of another and her story, in the time that's left, if you would move across the rest of Claire's life, taking in and understanding once again all the meaning and richness and significance of things that take place during the remaining years.

Client: We have another child, a son.

Therapist: And his name?

Client: I keep getting different names. First, I was going to say Daniel, after my father. Then, I see French names coming up. I think it was Daniel. I don't see that Joseph's ancestry was French—that somehow he came there, his family did when he was very young. So, yes, we did name him Daniel. They're adults now with children of their own. We've had a happy life, a successful life. We were never wealthy from our paintings, but we were happy and had plenty.

Therapist: That sounds like its own kind of wealth.

Client: That's right. We're slowing down now, as we're older. We still enjoy just walking in the countryside, whether it's just for the pleasure of the walk or to do our painting again. But now it's just for our own enjoyment—the painting is.

[*Her face flinches.*]

Therapist: What just happened?

Client: I see myself stumbling. We're out on one of those walks. It's very rocky, big rocks. I fell. Joseph is over me ... to see if I'm okay. I don't know. I'm hurt from the fall but I don't know how badly I'm hurt. I'm just lying on the ground. I can't walk so Joseph is very torn whether to leave me and get help or stay there. [*Again she flinches.*] I feel myself ... fading away ... it's all getting purple now. I feel above it.

Therapist: As you look at Claire's body, do you see any indications of injuries?

Client: I know the legs were injured or broken because she couldn't walk. That's why Joseph didn't know whether to go get help. I see my head on a rock. I don't feel that I'm totally dead, just sort of coming and going. One minute I'll feel myself and the next I feel I'm looking down on it. I'm trying to speak to Joseph but the words won't come out. He's very upset. He's picking my torso up and holding me, rocking me in his arms. I've died now. I see him just sitting there rocking me, holding me. He doesn't want to go for help right away. He just wants to spend some final time with me.

Therapist: [*Pause.*] When you're ready, I'd like to invite you, if you haven't already noticed the Light, to perhaps turn around and let yourself become aware of what is available to you in this time of transition, and would like to invite Claire and Dorothy to take this opportunity to meet. And as we have done before, to take advantage of this time to exchange even further observations, thoughts, decisions.

Client: I see Claire was allowed to look quietly down at Joseph for a while in the afternoon light, to give her time to say goodbye to him. She loved him deeply. When she's ready she turns around.

I'm waiting—just quietly waiting until she's ready. We embrace. She's sad to leave her life. But on the other hand, she had such a full life she doesn't have regrets. Now she's showing me where she fell and the back of her head that hit the rock. It's almost like she's saying it's the same place I'm hurt but she died from hers.

I see she's sorry she wasn't able to speak to Joseph after she hit her head. I see she was in and out of consciousness as she died … trying to fight against it to come back to him. When she's conscious that she's dying, things will just get grayer for her and darker as she lapses back into unconsciousness.

Therapist: If we might, let's check with her and if this needs the confirmation of others who may be in the background ready to assist her. Let's check to see if she would like to double-check what she brings with her from this life just completed and what she leaves with the physical body, so that she may choose clearly and wisely what she brings with her and what she leaves there with the body.

Client: She does bring her sorrow at not being able to communicate and sorrow that she died as quickly … that she didn't have time for her goodbyes.

Therapist: Did she make any decisions about that ... about what she would do different next time, if anything?

Client: No, she doesn't feel she needs to do anything different. They were a very loving family. It's just her sorrow of leaving them so quickly ... and unexpectedly.

Therapist: Would you check with her to make sure that in some way that in bringing that sorrow with her, which would certainly seem to make sense, that she is able to leave behind in the physical body those things which happened to it because of the fall, so that there with you her legs work well and she can walk freely with complete balance, even as she did in her youth and throughout so much of her adult life? [*Pause.*] And that she checks to make sure that with the sorrow that she brings with her ... and that ache ... that she leaves the physical injuries that occurred to the physical body there with that body. Bringing with her the clarity that she used in her paintings, the clarity that she used in developing her skills in being able to communicate in two written languages, as well as through her painting, so that in the body in which she stands there before you, she can know how free she is to retain all of that clarity and wisdom and ability to communicate in so many different ways, whether with movement, the brush on the canvas and the paper, or with words, or with images, so that she is both able to take in that which she sees, that which she hears, and the sense of movement, the body in space, and then use all of that information with such ease and speed and balance ... leaving with the physical body that which belongs with the physical body. Just as surely as she would have washed out her brushes to remove all the residue of paint when she was through at the easel so that the brush was clear and soft and flexible and clean and ready for its next use, so, too, with your help and those who are available to her, she can in this time enjoy washing the soul's body clean, so that at its deepest levels it is clear of any pigment from an earlier project that might impede its freedom in the future. And having assisted her in whatever way makes sense, if you are willing to invite her and all of those who are here for you also, to assist in a similar process ... washing out all that has served its purpose, cleaning the brush of this body, checking each fibre, each connection. And perhaps as a way of comparing and knowing how well that has been done ... that even when it is time for her to head off into the Light for her own rest and to await the time when Joseph likewise makes his transition, that the two of you, before she departs, might embrace once again ... and in that way that these things are able to be ... to take in all of the clarity and ability to think and process ... taking in and giving back, with her eyes, with her thoughts, with her words, with her movements ... that with that embrace and each breath in, to accept that gift from her as a remembrance of another time when your soul celebrated all that is possible using physical form ... just as she celebrated through her life what is possible with watercolors and Joseph with oils and knowing that she can look forward to the joy and creativity that your own way of expressing yourself has taken place and will continue to manifest in your own life. And, as always, to enjoy any gifts of her own observations that she may have for you.

Client: I see her telling me to start with a clean page ... to paint my own life and my own beauty ... with the softness and colors that I want. To go with my feelings ... to go with the happy and bright colors: the yellows and the blues, greens ... just a bit of purple. To feel free ... to express myself freely. It doesn't matter that I don't have her techniques ... just to paint what I feel ... that it doesn't take talent; it just takes emotion. I see her showing me the colors and shapes I would want, saying, "Just enjoy." It's like I see her sweeping her arm to the page I've painted that's now big and large ... covering our whole view ... saying, "Now go paint the rest of your life."

Therapist: Any other messages that she has for you or those who may be there with you before she takes her leave today?

Client: I do feel others around. I feel she was taking her leave as we were looking at this painting ... at my painting of my life. That she was leaving me as she was saying, "To paint my own life ahead ... to paint it as I want it to be ... to be happy."

Therapist: She seems to have understood how happiness is a by-product of choices.

Client: Yes. Yes, I feel that just in the choices I am making in my own life today how much calmer, happier, at peace I feel. Glad I've taken control again.

Therapist: So allowing time for any additional messages and with each breath in taking in all that is true about this for you now, [*pausing to pace her exhale*] with each breath out releasing all that has served its function, all that is no longer true ... like washing the residual pigment from the brush, leaving it clean for the next time at the easel, choosing whichever color, whichever shape, whichever content and topic is right for that time ... each time ... and when all of that is stored deeply within, and the feelings associated with that radiate throughout your truth ... with that clarity of thought and mind

and body and soul, becoming clearer with each breath, each
moment, let your eyes open again.

Dorothy's series of waking dreams correlated with a marked shift
in her mood. Her depression was gone and she felt much more opti-
mistic about her ability to deal with her life. She had also become
more comfortable allowing others to help her at times. Her sense of
autonomy no longer precluded asking others for assistance. At a
follow up nearly two years after her first appointment, she noted
that her neurological symptoms continued to be much improved.
Perhaps even more importantly, she again commented on the
enduring qualitative changes in her life. She continued to draw on
the love and support from Claire and George and her father.
Whenever she pulled back too far into her shell, they were there
encouraging her to keep reaching out to those around her.

I would like to say that her story ends there, but about five years
after her first appointment with me, she developed cancer. She
resumed therapy with me as she confronted this new challenge.
Eventually, the tumor became metastatic and resistant to further
treatment. Shortly before she died, she remarked how her earlier
work had provided her with the strength to face even this challenge, to live each day fully and enjoy the love and support she
received from her family and friends.

Chapter 5
We Make it Harder than it Needs to Be

Matthew

One of the common applications of waking dreams is in helping clients identify faulty assumptions that have kept them stuck in some way. On occasion, I use this story with one of my clients to demonstrate how faulty assumptions can lead to a belief that there is no solution to a problem.

> One evening at our local hospital an ambulance crew brought in a 16-year-old boy who had been in a car accident. From the boy's pale skin color it was easy to see that he had lost considerable blood. The attending physician quickly assessed that the accident had caused significant internal bleeding and told the hospital staff to get the boy prepped for surgery. Then the physician told the staff to page Dr. Johnson, adding, "I can't perform the surgery because this boy is my son." The physician, however, was not the boy's father. Who was the physician? [The answer is in the footnote below.]

The waking dream that follows is from a middle-aged male, Matthew, who had grown up with the belief that women possess "magic" and men do not. Therefore, he believed that in order to have access to it, a man has to be close to a woman. As a result, when he found himself between relationships, he experienced

---

*If one makes the *faulty* assumption that all physicians are males, there is no solution to this "problem". Many people do not even realize, however, that they have made such an assumption. Once the person allows for the possibility that physicians can be men *or* women, the "problem" disappears, as the physician is obviously the boy's mother. (If you tell the story to others, be sure to use a *male* patient to bias the exception that the story is about males. Fewer people get stuck if the patient is a female.)

considerable anxiety. He had good insight into some likely origins for this belief, but that had not been enough to resolve his anxiety when he was between relationships.

In his waking dream, Matthew experienced himself as a nun, Antoinette, who lived her life in a convent. Even as a child, Antoinette had understood that her father was afraid of power and of misusing it. He had brought her to the convent, in part, so that she might pray for family fortune, the success of people close to him, and the like. As might be expected, her early memories of the convent were of feeling excluded from the world outside. Referring to other teenagers, she said, "They are allowed out of the cell, this room, and I am not."

As the dream continued, Matthew reported a major shift: the young woman had experienced separation as a kind of exile, but suddenly had the experience "that God missed me". Matthew periodically interjected his own observations about correlations between physiological aspects of the hypnotic experience and memories of some of the Psalms from the Old Testament that had long held meaning for him. As he experienced being the nun, he described a kinesthetic sense of his throat area knowing what was true ("love"), as contrasted with his mouth area ("fear"), which he described as trying to dismiss what he was experiencing. He reported being quite moved by the parallels between his emotional reactions to the old Psalms, the young nun's emotional experiences as she prayed, and his own physical reactions. In this context, Antoinette commented at one point, "All songs are the same song."

When I asked if he was willing "to explore the rest of [Antoinette's] life," Matthew briefly reported about the tone of the nun's adult life, and then had a spontaneous OBE experience following her death. The nun, who had since become the Mother Superior of the convent, found herself talking with Jesus and Mother Mary. In a dialogue involving himself, Antoinette, and the other two, Matthew reported further insights. He had seen magic as something external to himself; something you go find and then get incorporated by it. As Antoinette, Matthew had had the experience of creating a space *within himself* into which the magic could enter. He also suddenly had the realization that power is just another form of magic. Taken together, these insights served to shatter Matthew's faulty assumption that only women could have magic (i.e., power). As he internalized these experiences and insights, he reported being "flooded with light". Following the trance work, he commented about the power of the contrasts of the two religious traditions, but even more so about the masculine-feminine contrast. He commented again about the "Aha!" shift from perceiving power as something external to something internal.

Here is the transcript of Matthew's waking dream:

Therapist: What can we focus on at this particular place?

Client: I want to focus on a present life phenomenon that goes in my formulation, "It's as if I have this magical belief that women possess magic. Men in general, and I in specific, don't. And therefore I have to have a woman close to me in order to be close to 'manna' as it were." Now what I cognitively know about it is that it would fit with literal stories my mother would tell me. Her specific variant would be, "She was magical, loved me and did in a way that no one else could ever love me, including me; and men were a bunch of idiots who couldn't cross the streets by themselves." It fits with my preschool years after my parents divorced. My parents divided the kids and my brother was my dad's and I was my mother's. My mother agrees with this by the way. That's what I know about it cognitively. What I know emotionally is I seem to go into a panic if I am in a status without a woman—like unmarried. When I was in college, I wrote a piece about, "Oh my God! I don't have a date on Friday night and what does this mean?" There's a piece of me that still thinks that. A piece of me that still believes that is true, [*that*] somehow I am being, in a major way, judged and found wanting.

Therapist: Okay, ready to go? [*He nods.*] In some counties today is the last day of school, and parents and children alike are celebrating in all the different ways what that means—to have reached another milestone—another transition point. It will be commencement for some, an ending, and yet it's called a beginning—a time when we get to look forward and yet enjoy looking back savoring all that we've learned and all that we've experienced. And in sorting out all that we will take with us and what we will leave behind in so many ways that may be both conscious and sometimes otherwise, making decisions about what is true based on those experiences, and what is no longer true and can be left behind with that period of life ... And so it is that just as coral in the ocean is built up layer upon layer, the rocks deep within the Earth are added to layer upon layer. So, too, it seems we build the wisdom of the soul through so many of these experiences across time.

Different kinds of relationships, different in age, different in gender, different in the nature of the intimacy, different in the gifts that each brings, and just as the adult can watch the child exploring something new and somehow seeing in the child's eyes *life as if it is magical* ... [*each word spoken more slowly, beginning to reframe life rather than women as* "magical".] ... and remembering somewhere deep within how it must have been true for us at some point, that we can recognize that sense of awe and wonder and joy in the child who touches and experiences that magic.

I continue toying with the connotations Matthew has long attached to "magic" by implicitly inviting him to view the world through a child's eyes as something "magical". The references to transitions above and those that follow were intended to subtly convey the idea that his own beliefs about magic could also be in transition.

Therapist: Today might be a wonderful time as people are in transition and moving from one way of being to another, each in their own way, to travel across time and space, to a story that will add another level of meaning and understanding to your beliefs about what magic is, who has it, how it is acquired, how it is used, and other assumptions about that which children seem to know and understand. And as adults, like we forget how we learned how to ride a bicycle, sometimes we forget what we learned about magic. And as that story begins to emerge and take form as a thought ... or a feeling ... an image ... a body sensation, let me know what you find ...

Client: A tightening in my chest, a beginning of ... tearing. A resistance to the tearing [*crying*], and I can see a light blue sky.

Therapist: Given that the sky is a light blue that would suggest that the sun is up in the sky today.

Client: Uh-huh.

Therapist: Would it be okay if some of the warmth and love of that sunlight came down to that place that feels tight? To breathe the gift of life into that place so that both can work their magic. Father-son and Mother-Earth coming together to create enough space to hold gently whenever that tightness and those tears are about ...

Client: There is a window that has either leaded glass or … I don't know if I see bars across it or like I read the description in a book that says that it has bars across it. Now I'm confused because I know I'm staring at a page in a novel about a French saint who lives in a room like this all her life, so I'm not sure if I'm seeing it or scanning the page or both.

Therapist: Okay.

Client: But I have a kinesthetic of—there is an experience in the big world that lots of people can have from which I'm excluded.

Therapist: Do you know what that experience is?

Client: No, but I think it's on the other side of the window. It's like, they are all out, out of the cell, the room, and I'm not. I don't know what the experience is.

Therapist: Would be important to know more about where you are as a frame of reference?

Client: I don't know.

Therapist: If it would be important to know more about how it is that you come to be in this room or this cell, or what it is to be here, that might begin to unfold … Or if not, to focus on what it is you see outside that is in such contrast to what you experience inside this room …

Client: There's a room which is pretty dark, and there's a much lighter space over here [*he gestures*], but I don't know what's happening in the lighted space. All I can see is there is more light there.

Therapist: Okay. And where are you in relationship to those?

Client: I'm here looking that way [*he gestures*]. The window faces that way. I don't know how in God's name I see light over here.

Therapist: Are these separate rooms here, or different spaces of the same room?

Client: I'm not even sure this is a room. It may be a courtyard.

Therapist: Okay. And is there some kind of a door between them?

Client: There is a door out of the cell, but I haven't been outside the cell for so long, I don't know where it goes.

Therapist: Do you know if the door can be opened from where you are?

Client: The door can be opened from the outside, not from the inside …

Therapist: When you look out the window can you see just sky, or can you see ground?

Client: I currently don't see ground.

Therapist: Okay. As you look about this room what else do you see that would identify what functions this room serves for you?

Client: It's got a place to pray. Oh lordy, lordy. All right! Again, this may be the book, but it certainly has the feel of a cell in a monastery or nunnery. It's got a *prie dieu*, it's got a …

Therapist: Have you noticed what gender you are?

Client: I'm tempted to say female, but again, I'm tempted by the book, but my hunch is female. The room has a statue of the Virgin, a blue and white statue …

Therapist: And if it's important, notice how old you seem to be.

Client: The words that come into my head are 16 …

Therapist: How long have you been at this place?

Client: Since somewhere between five and eight.

Therapist: Is it important to know how you came to be at such a place at that age?

Client: My father took me there. I'm not clear if voluntarily. .

Therapist: What do know about his decision to bring you there, if it's important.

Client: I have two intuitions about it. One, that it was political. The other is that he sensed I had a talent for prayer, and he thought that was important and it frightened him. And it wasn't real world important, but it frightened him.

Therapist: What about prayer would be something that he would call a talent in the sense of doing things with talents?

Client: I could pray for the family fortune. I could pray for the success of people close to him. I could ask God to forgive him.

Therapist: Does he need forgiveness? Did he think he did?

Client: Yes, he thought he did.

Therapist: Do know what that was about?

Client: Intuitively, there was some political stuff he was ashamed of. I know it's sinful. [*Here, Matthew comments as an aside,* "Is it dissociative if I think, 'I got this from an opera; I got this from a book?'"]

Therapist: It's a good way for the conscious mind to be skeptical about how to interpret it.

Client: Okay.

Therapist: It's a way of keeping it at arm's length.

Client: I could do a running commentary on which opera, which book, but I figured that was boring.

Therapist: I would invite your left brain to enjoy the ways in which this story has so many parallels to that literature, and how that may make the story one which indeed has components which are timeless and archetypical. And is it willing to allow the rest of self to experience the timelessness and meaning of these themes, knowing that it has the rest of this lifetime and certainly beyond, to explore analytical interpretations of these things?

Matthew recognized that he could spend a lot of time wondering about possible sources for the imagery he was experiencing. My suggestion was intended to acknowledge and honor his curiosity and skepticism in a way that would enable him to postpone his analysis of the waking dream until he had finished having it.

Client: Oh, okay. Sure. [*Pause.*] He [*Antoinette's father*] has done and will continue to do things political that he knows are sinful, and he thinks they are necessary.

Therapist: At 16, what are other girls typically doing?

Client: At 16, they would be raising their children. Or they would be in court, or they would be managing an estate.

Therapist: Would they also be outside?

Client: Obviously. Or be in court, technically on the outside.

Therapist: What else is it that the people outside this window are allowed to do, to be or to have, that you find yourself drawn to but unable to get to because of where you are?

Client: They can walk wherever they want. [*Pause.*] They don't have to bear their parents' ... okay ... two sentences: They don't have to bear their parents' obsessive burdens, and they don't have to bear God's incessant demands.

Therapist: Okay.

Client: And I don't know. [*Pause.*] I confuse the two.

Therapist: Um-hmm.

Client: Sometimes I have the sense that God ... [*Pause.*] Sometimes I have a sense that God demanded loving. I don't have a sense that my father did. They both have that incessant quality, an implacable, overwhelming quality.

Therapist: Is God's loving demand that God demands that you love, or is it that God's demand comes in a loving way, or is there a difference?

Client: The content of what God demands is that I use my talent to pray; that He gave me that talent and that is what I should do. But, yes, the content of the prayer: [*Pause.*] to pray perfectly I should love perfectly. At seconds I feel that love, and that almost convinces me I'm not too envious of the world outside. I don't miss it.

Therapist: Is it possible that the experience of both allows a deeper appreciation of both? The more that you miss that which is outside, the more you can appreciate the experience of that love and contentment?

Client: Hmmmm, I never thought of it that way. I intuit it as possible. My throat says it is possible. This part of my body [*he gestures to his throat*] says it's possible. Actually, this [*his throat*] part of my body says it knows what you said is true.

Therapist: Okay.

Client: There's another part of my body that says this is the kind of crap that people tell me.

Therapist: Which part? [*He gestures to his mouth.*] Would you invite the two to take in a large breath, and there in the Light of the room to dialogue with each other, whether in words or in experience, about those contrasting beliefs and feelings.

Client: [*Long pause with a big sigh when he exhales.*]

Therapist: … and I would start with the interesting premise that both are true.

Client: Of course.

Therapist: That it's not a question of "either—or", but how can both be true? What is one to do with that reality that indeed both are true if that is true?

Client: … We've had the dialogue … The envy and the sadness create more space for the love to enter. Yeah, I didn't ask for this, and I don't like it, and it's not what I would have wanted. God's voice, "Yeah, I didn't get what I asked for either." "You didn't?" "No, I didn't." At which point it synthesized, calmed down, and my breathing shifted.

Therapist: It sounds like the mouth stopped viewing the throat as an enemy who betrayed the mouth.

Client: And there was something very moving, and the mouth read it as an invitation from God to help God grow. I was moved by that, [*Pause.*] that God missed me, was longing for me.

Therapist: I don't know if at 16 you had yet had a chance to study the Old Testament as much as might be true about the New

Testament. The mouth seems to have held some anger at a kind of betrayal that many a person thinks in a New Testament way that it's not okay to be angry with God. I'm struck with the simple dichotomy of the mouth and throat, the Old Testament and New, of a fearful God and a loving God, and an invitation that could exist for a re-connection of those aspects to grow in discovering that the oneness of self really wasn't a betrayal—to reconnect with the part of self that has been missed for a time. And in the metaphor, to reconnect with the God that has missed us. To allow not only the throat to feel that love, but to risk allowing the mouth to feel the love. To challenge the belief perhaps: whether feeling the love requires surrendering anger permanently, or just allowing balance.

Client: Right. I had accepted the separation as an exile …

Therapist: What are you now calling that separation?

Client: A space between. In the image of the Psalm, the Shepherd calling his sheep …

Therapist: And indeed, the mouth and the throat and the lungs and the heart must work together if the Shepherd is going to call out loud to the sheep. The absence of any one makes that experience impossible.

Client: Mmmm!

Therapist: And what sound would this girl's mouth and throat and lungs and heart make if they took in a breath of life and used that God-given talent to utter a statement of prayer?

Client: In the Old Testament they would blow the shofar. In the New they would utter Mary's Magnificat, "My soul doth magnify the Lord."

Therapist: If you'd like, take a moment to experience that internally, to let her pray in the way that she has come to learn the prayer. To be her. *To feel the magic.* [*Long pause.*] And let me know when you've reached the "Amen".

Client: … Okay.

Therapist: Anything about that that you would share?

Client: The light moved to the inside of the cell. God was in the cell. Bach was right: the Lord invites you to the heavenly feast. Every feast is the heavenly feast. And there's probably a way in which all songs are the same song. That's an inference from when you said, "Tell me when you get to the 'Amen'."

Therapist: Okay.

Client: I hear this singer singing Arthur Sullivan's The Lost Chord which ends up with, "It may be only in heaven that I shall hear that grand 'Amen'." And then a thought that went, "But every place is heaven."

Therapist: For if indeed the Lord is everywhere and everything, how could the Lord *not* be in this room? [*Intentional ambiguity about which room—the cell or my office.*]

Client: Right.

Therapist: Except that we might forget to notice, or choose not to. For there are some like the father who is afraid of what the talent might mean, and how his own life might change if he were to really touch and know the power of that talent. [*Pause.*]

Without specifically naming the client as one of the "some", the pause was intended to let him linger with the experience he has just had as the nun touching/knowing the power of that talent. The verb choice "if he were" implies he hasn't, but he actually had touched it, thus making the life changes more possible.

Therapist: Would it be useful to notice how the rest of this girl's life proceeds?

Client: Um-hmm. I'm certainly curious about it.

Therapist: Let's take a few moments to do a survey of the major points across her life span … And let me know when you've reached the end of it … Or anything else important that you want to share …

Client: [*Long pause.*] I see her living and flourishing. I don't see her dying. [*Pause.*] Wrong.

Therapist: Okay. Notice the circumstances [pause] and notice any final thoughts that occur [*pause*] and moving through the experience of death, its own commencement [*returning to the theme that I introduced during the induction about endings and beginnings*] … enjoying an opportunity to complete a review of this life now finished, whether that is done individually or in the presence of those who are here to assist in that journey into the Light ... And when that feels complete, let me know, as I have a request.

Client: [*Pause.*] Okay.

Therapist: I would like to invite who she has been and who you are, perhaps in a split screen view of her life and your life, to notice whatever else is relevant about the theme of "magic" and gender beliefs about who has it and how it is acquired.

Client: [*Long pause.*]

Therapist: And if it would be okay with you, who happens to have been male in this lifetime, to experience your own magic just as you have experienced hers, except in a way that works for you in this body and space and time.

Client: She smiles ...

Therapist: And to check out any faulty assumptions you may have had until now [*I'm implying the faulty assumptions have now been recognized and released*] ... about how it feels to experience the magic yourself.

Client: Okay.

Therapist: And then notice how the two of you would like to bring this to a close ... if there is anything else to check ... parallels between her lifetime and yours ... people who may seem to have been present in both ... and when that is complete, with each breath, enjoying the knowledge that, taking in and storing all that is true and useful about this for you, releasing with each breath any assumption that no longer fits ... and knowing how many different ways the soul, the body, the mind can express the feelings, the knowledge, the wisdom, the love that has come out over the centuries as song, as prayer, as an infinite variety of "Amens". And taking all about this that is true for you, to re-orient to this time and place ... looking forward to the ways that this, too, will become manifest in the days and weeks ahead, till when that is done you can let your eyes open again ...

I like to close hypnosis work with some standard suggestions that help the person (a) let go of assumptions that were found to be incorrect, (b) hold on to that which seems true, and (c) have an expectation that positive changes from this work will take place in the coming weeks.

Client: [*Opens his eyes and grins.*] That is hysterical, hysterical! Parts of it were so funny! There is a Marx Brothers quality to it. She dies. She's a Mother Superior by now. She's watching her nuns anxiously praying for her. The other side of death is so wonderfully playful, that she is sort of—it's not quite dancing. It's like floating with Mary and Jesus to this music from the Mahler 8th [*Symphony*] in which these spirits of Heaven are sung by a boys' choir and she looks at Mary and says, "You mean it was always this easy!?" And Mary goes, [*client is laughing*] "Yeah, but nobody gets it." And she looks at Jesus and says, "Was it always this easy for you?" And Jesus says, "Yea, but nobody gets its." It's funny.

Therapist: I'm curious about what happened in the final dialogues that the two of you had about magic and your initial question.

Client: What she saw earlier, so we had shared it before the final dialogue, what she saw earlier was—it's a kinesthetic experience, how the hell do I put it into words … okay—I, Matthew, the directionality I had was, "Magic is external to me. You go out of yourself towards it, grab something outside of yourself, and try to get incorporated *by* it."

Therapist: Get incorporated *by* it? So you have to go there and get incorporated by the other?

Client: Yes. She found that God has to subtract from Himself to create an emptiness into which the magic can enter. The cabalistic statement is, "God created nothing in order for there to be a space into which He could enter." God subtracted from Himself. What she got was a kinesthetic of, "You let God into you. That creates a space into which the magic enters." The magic is an energy exchange between you and God—to be prosaic about it.

Therapist: Did you then get that in a kinesthetic way?

Client: Oh, yeah. Oh, yeah. I was flooded with light. "She" was flooded with light technically.

When you asked me to look for people in the nun's life I realized I couldn't … I knew the father in the girl's story was a parent in my life, but I didn't know which one. Still don't. But then I had a set of thoughts that went, "Oh, if it's my father, and he really had this kind of power, what I saw then was a man who was so afraid of how he would misuse power that he wasn't going to let himself have any." And that's stupid. Power is just another form of magic. You don't have to be consumed by it. It's another form of energy. It's not that big a deal.

… She [*the nun*] is right about the Psalms.

Therapist: For whatever reason, I was remembering where the Psalms invoke the freedom to invoke anger, to be really angry at God, to really call Him on the carpet, and how that just doesn't fit with what many believe about the New Testament; that in the New Testament you don't get angry at God.

Client: What that did for me, what I did with it, is I went, "Okay. Now in subsequent questions I can do a Jewish answer and a Christian answer. This is cool. This is integrative."

Therapist: [*Discussing the imagery of the Shepherd*] who calls out because not only is he responsible for the sheep, but he loves them.

Client: That's right. Exactly. And that was the image. That was the shift in me about … Ahhh! This is relevant actually. Two years ago, a woman told me something which I heard, and knew she was absolutely right, but didn't know what to do with it. She said that I confused loneliness with missing God. The nun had the experience [*of the loneliness*], which is why I said I thought I was in exile. It's only a separation. I got it! That's where I got the shepherd from. "Oh! He's been waiting for me to come back! I thought I was like being put in 'time out,' and He has to take me out of time out."

In closing, Matthew noted that the greater intensity for him was not the religious contrast, but the gender contrast.

In a follow-up meeting with Matthew about two years later, he commented on a significant shift in his life that had subsequently taken place where religion and spirituality were concerned. Having shed the faulty assumption that power is something that has to be found externally, his personal life had moved in new directions with which he was very pleased.

Chapter 6
"But I Don't See Anything"

Eric

New clients come with a variety of expectations and preconceived ideas about what they hope will happen or think "should" happen with hypnosis. Those who have prior experience with hypnosis or various forms of meditation often move easily into a hypnotic state. For most, visual imagery comes as quickly as it does in nighttime dreams, typically accompanied by other sensory experiences, such as sounds and tactile sensations. A small percentage of new clients report that, "I don't see anything" after a few minutes in trance. When this happens, it usually means I missed something while I was getting background information about the person. In most cases, this can be resolved after some questioning to ascertain what is meant by "nothing".

I have found there are four common reasons for this kind of initial difficulty:

1. A few clients are so eager to begin that they have trouble relaxing enough.

This is analogous to trying to make yourself fall asleep. To go to sleep, you must be willing to turn over control to a different part of your own mind/body. Trance, while very different from sleep, involves the same paradox: going into trance requires a willingness to let a different part of your mind/soul become active. Unlike sleep, though, your conscious mind can resume "control" whenever it wants during trance. Think of how breathing works. Any time you want you can choose to breathe in a different way. Yet as soon as you forget to remember to breathe consciously, some other part of your mind/body immediately takes over the task of monitoring your breathing.

When clients seem too eager, I walk them through a more structured initial sequence that may begin with a focus on more external events, such as awareness of different parts of the body, of breathing, of sounds coming from outside my office, etc. Gradually, I mix these with awareness of internal thoughts or memories of recent events. Alternatively, I may ask clients to describe a place and time when they felt very relaxed, very safe, and very comfortable. Most of this group can recreate this kind of memory easily, in part because they don't equate doing so with "being in trance".

2. Some clients have prior histories involving violations of trust.

This is particularly so when there has been a history of trauma or abuse. Because the common, though faulty, belief is that the client relinquishes control to the therapist when in trance, such clients often simply need more time to accomplish two critical tasks: First, they need more time to decide whether they trust the therapist. Second, they need time to discover that they, themselves, control whether or not they go into trance, and if so, to what level. Years ago, I demonstrated this for one client with the help of a colleague. I explained that after I helped the colleague go into trance, I would signal to the client so that she could ask any questions she wanted of my colleague—who would remain in trance. In this way, she was able to see what it looked like to be "in trance" and was able to satisfy her fears and curiosities about the illusion of control. Next, I invited the woman to go in and out of trance several times with the colleague still in the room. In this way, she was able to test for herself what she had just observed with my colleague.

3. Some clients initially report difficulty because what is happening doesn't match their expectations.

While I was doing some research a few years ago, one of the volunteers, Eric, reported for three straight sessions that "nothing is happening". At the end of the third session, he finally revealed that he had had lots of images, but he had rejected every one of them because he thought he was "making them up". To his surprise, I asked him to intentionally do just that: make up a scene. He immediately began reporting rich imagery that was quite relevant to core issues in his life at that time. The waking dream that ensued is presented later in this chapter.

4. A fourth small group has trouble with hypnotic (visual) imagery because these clients work best in a different sensory channel.

Some people deal with auditory or tactile (kinesthetic) information better than they deal with visual information. For these people, I find it easiest to shift my language to their preferred sensory channel. Imagine that instead of staring at a blank TV screen waiting for an image to appear you put on headphones and turn on the radio. Instead of asking, "What do you see as you look around?" I may say, "Notice if you hear a voice or any other sounds," or, "Notice any thoughts that come into your awareness." For those who find it easier to deal with feelings and tactile sensations, I may say, "Notice any changes in how your body feels; whether one arm feels warmer or heavier ..." Or if the person has been to the beach, I may suggest the person return there and, "Notice how it feels to walk along the sand. Notice if the sand feels wet or dry ... whether there is a breeze blowing ... the warmth of the sun." Once I understand which sensory channels work best for this kind of person, it becomes an easy matter to use matching language to facilitate his or her waking dreams.

The waking dream that follows was reported by Eric, the middle-aged, married man who had responded to an ad I had placed in a local newspaper for hypnosis research subjects. His marriage of many years had been in a long, slow decline that seemed to have evolved into a death spiral. I think he "knew" it was only a matter of time before he filed for a divorce, but he was not yet ready to take the finality of that step.

Once Eric got over his surprise that I would ask him to "make up" an image, he generated his first image, a rich multi-sensory one, within seconds. Buoyed by that experience, we concluded that session, his third, on a positive note. The following week, I invited him to begin as he had done at the close of the previous session, by intentionally making up an image. The imagery in the resulting waking dream provided a powerful metaphor for his "dead" marriage:

> **Therapist:** Take a minute, relax and go inside, and at some point, just like we did at the end of the session last time, generate an image. Whether you think of something on purpose or it just happens to be there. Let me know and we'll go from there.

Client: I was intrigued with the road. [*This was part of the image he had had at the end of the previous session.*] I was thinking about it a good bit this week. Kind of an interesting reaction to it. I kept thinking about the road and wanting to go down that road to see what was down there, but not wanting to do it during the week by myself. Every time I was thinking about it I thought, "Oh, no, no. Don't do it now!" So I thought I'd wait until the session.

Therapist: Let's go back to the road. As I remember it was a dirt road that forked, and you clearly wanted to take the left fork which shortly after went around a curve.

Here I take a minute to help him re-establish the imagery and elaborate on it. By doing this, he was able to deepen his trance effortlessly without realizing it.

Client: That's right. I couldn't look down the road because it curved and was blocked by trees. I was walking down this road dressed in boots and long pants and a long sleeve, baggy, cotton shirt.

Therapist: Anything on your head?

Client: I was just thinking about that. A straw hat. Something to keep the sun off. Something maybe a farmer would wear.

Therapist: Any sense of the time of year?

Client: Summer. Definitely summer. Hot. In fact I was thinking about the shirt being heavy because of how hot it was. But then thinking it was helping keep me cool. So I was thinking about warm temperatures. There's a dead tree right in the center of this road, like a big, old, oak tree that has died—been dead for quite a long time. The fork in this road is more or less—can see it a little clearer now—where the road goes straight and this is like a little turnoff from the main road. So it's not so much a fork as taking a little detour that curves away from the road off to the left and heads off into a more wooded area. I visualize it being open straight ahead, and the road to the left curving into a wooded area.

His language offers some rich metaphors about an alternative way of understanding what has been happening in his marriage. Rather than having to choose which course to take at a fork in the road, what lies to the left is a "little detour" into a wooded area. In dream imagery, going underwater or into a cave or wooded area are images that often translate as exploring one's inner self.

Therapist: Okay. Does the oak tree seem familiar?

After dealing with what he could see, I began to inquire about what he was feeling. Notice his sense of apprehension that begins to emerge.

Client: Not really. Familiar in the sense I've seen oak trees like that before.

Therapist: But as the person that you are on this dirt road, is there any sense of this tree being a familiar reference point?

Client: No I don't think so.

Therapist: Are you ready to walk down this side road?

Client: I think so [hesitantly]. Last week I think I mentioned I was, I had a feeling of anticipation. But right now I feel apprehensive about going down. I don't know why I feel differently. Maybe that's what I was feeling during the week when I was thinking about it. Maybe I didn't want to do it because I was a little apprehensive about it. [*It is very normal to have some apprehension when one contemplates probing the depths of the mind/soul/personality!*]

Therapist: Okay.

Client: So I'm kind of standing there on this dirt road. I'm on the left turn. I see the oak tree just in front of me to the right. I'm just standing there. The oak tree being, it looks rather forlorn. This big beautiful tree that's now dead. There are no leaves on it. Gives a feeling to the scene of sadness … Hasn't rained for a long time. I get the sense it's really hot and dry. It hasn't rained in a really long time. The road is really dusty. When I walk it kicks up a lot of powdery dirt.

Therapist: As you notice the dryness and that forlorn sense of this huge old oak tree that one time must have been so full of color and shade and vitality, notice if that serves as a stepping off point for reminiscing about something from this person's past, analogous to the implied history of this oak tree. The oak tree can't be this large and dead if it wasn't at some point this large and alive. So it must have a history. Is there anything about this person's history that is implied or hinted at by this oak tree and the sadness of this scene?

Client: I don't know. The only feeling I get is that the scene … it's almost as if the oak tree represents the dry conditions. It's really dry and hot. There's no water, not much water. Maybe the tree has died because of that. Maybe there's a correlation between this drought-like feeling about it and the dead tree.

Therapist: As you stand there on this dry powdery dirt road, do you have any sense of whether you are in a drought period emotionally —the man standing there in the road?

Client: It's not that I don't have a good feeling about this, but I don't know about *that* ...

Therapist: I think last week there was a dog that appeared. He had a name. Notice if that seems to fit this week or not.

Client: I didn't feel he was standing there with me.

Therapist: Would you like to walk far enough down this side road to be able to see around the trees that block the view?

Client: Yeah, yeah. The trees are blocking the view, but they're kind of stunted. They're not very tall. More like small trees and shrubs. As I walk along I can see on the side of the road tall grass that's covered in dust as if the wind had kicked up and coated the grass with the dusty earth. You can tell by looking at it that it's been a long time since there was any rain here. So I walk around this bend. It's a real gradual bend.

Therapist: Are you a male?

Client: Yeah.

Therapist: How old do you seem?

Client: Not too old. Maybe in my thirties or something like that. I turn around and look back on the big oak tree. I think I feel real upset that the tree has died. This is strange. I turn back and as I walk around this bend I get a picture of the road straightening out and going somewhat uphill in the distance and seeing a stormy sky up ahead. The way it gets when the dark clouds are rolling in but there's still bright light underneath them. Then you get this ridge of dark clouds up above so you can see this band of light below. That's the way it looks off in the distance up above this hill. Somehow I'm thinking at one level I should be really happy about this because it's really dry and maybe we're going to get some rain. But for some reason I don't feel that way. It doesn't really bring much pleasure. [*There are nice* *parallels here to his marriage—both in the past and in the near future.*]

Therapist: And I would invite you to simply let those feelings be there, even though they are not fully congruent with the thoughts. The feelings simply are there, and in time more may become clear about that. For now, maybe it's enough to be aware of how you feel in response to what you see as you go down this road … Are you still walking?

Many people have a tendency to dismiss *what* they're feeling if they do not understand *why* they are feeling that way. I didn't want him to get stuck analyzing the incongruities. Instead, I suggested that for now he take a more passive role and be aware of whatever he felt.

Client: I think I've come to—on the right side of the road—I've come to um … Somebody was living here, but they're not living here any more. It's a small house. Looks real broken down. There's a fence in front of the house. A small low picket fence maybe three feet high, but it's in disrepair. A lot of the pickets are broken out. There's a gate, but the gate's bent off the hinges. On the other side of this fence there's a garden, like somebody's vegetable garden, but it's all grown up with weeds and stuff. No one has lived here for quite awhile.

Therapist: Do you have a sense that you knew who lived here?

Client: Yeah, I was just thinking about it. I do feel like I knew somebody who lived there. I think it was a family. There's a sadness about this house, too. This whole scene is very sad. Something may have happened in the house. Some tragedy. Some unfortunate circumstance. I get the feeling someone just picked up and left kind of quickly and just left it all behind.

Therapist: Is there a sense that the whole family did that?

Client: The whole family did that. They had young children … One of them died.

Therapist: Boy or girl?

Client: I think it was a boy. He fell into a well. I can see the well off to the left front of the house.

Therapist: How ironic that the boy died from something that now is in such short supply.

Client: That's true. Yeah, he wasn't that old. He was only seven or eight years old. I'm not sure why they left this house. I don't know if it was because of the child dying. There's a real sadness to this house though. Real sad.

Therapist: Is there something you would like to do for this house? Or is this house more a part of a sequence in proceeding down this road?

Client: I'm not sure. I feel like I have some connection to the house. Like I was a good friend to some of the people that lived there, because I feel this sense of loss, sadness, because of what happened there. It's pretty lonely; I'm getting this really lonely feeling. There's nobody else around. I'm starting to get this feeling I'm all by myself. It's part of the feeling of this whole scene—there seems to be nobody else around but me ... I guess there's nothing left there at the house. I just stopped and now I think I'm going to walk along the road some more. I still see the hill up ahead and the sky with the brightness underneath and the darkness on the top ... I feel that I wish the house was back the way it used to be in happier times. It was a real pretty little house and well cared for. Small, but had a warm feel to it. There was happiness there.

Therapist: Sometimes at a funeral there is a ritual performed by all those in attendance where they place a rock or some dirt or something else symbolic on the fresh grave as a way of making an acknowledgment that what was special about this person is no longer available in physical form. That which brought the happiness and the joy and pleasure is no longer there. That ritual is a way of acknowledging what is. Notice if it feels right as you leave to place a stone or some dirt or something that you might have in a pocket, or to scratch something in the sand that would function as that way of acknowledging that that which used to be in happier times no longer inhabits this place, and that like the oak tree it now feels devoid of that which gave it life. In your parting you are acknowledging that which is.

One important aspect of grieving any kind of loss is to be willing to consciously accept that the loss has occurred. To do so does not require that we condone or excuse what happened that caused the loss, simply that it has occurred. As Frank Zappa once said, "Reality is what it is, not what we want it to be." If the man's marital home is as devoid of life as the house in his imagery, it is important that he acknowledges that reality.

> **Client:** For some reason, I have a knife in my pocket, an old, folding jackknife I feel like leaving there. It may have belonged to somebody in the house. I think it belonged to the child. He gave it to me for some reason. Seems strange I'd want to leave it there.

> **Therapist:** Does it seem like it's time to move on?

> **Client:** Yea, I guess.

> **Therapist:** Is that as much as not being sure you want to go forward or about not being sure that you're done here?

> **Client:** Yea, I think I'm still not sure about walking forward. Sort of like I'm just lingering there.

> **Therapist:** When you came to the old oak tree there was a clear decision about whether to take the left fork or go straight on down the road. Notice as you stand in front of the house at the edge of the road if it seems to make sense to go to the right or the left.

> **Client:** I definitely don't want to go back where I came from. I don't want to turn back. I really wish this man hadn't left. It's like there's a real sense of loss and loneliness … They may, the reason ... they may have left because of this drought. I feel this dry period was very long. It's been several years and all his crops had died and he was unable to live there any more …

> **Therapist:** If it would be important, notice how you have survived in this place when he and his family could not.

Here I am exploring his awareness of other resources that are available to him in the dream imagery that may have parallels in his day-to-day life. His response, however, reflects the sense of mental numbing characteristic of his way of talking about his current life circumstances.

> **Client:** I don't know how I have survived or why I'm still there. I do feel that in this immediate area where I am that there aren't many people left.

Therapist: When he left, apparently he took what was left of his family. Do you have any sense of whether you have family or relatives?

Client: I was trying to think of that a little bit ago. I feel like I'm alone. … Hmmm … I'm okay. I was just trying to think if I'm sick or really hungry, but physically I'm fine. In fact I seem to be a fairly large, muscular person … One thing I noticed about this house and every place I've gone, is that there's no, I don't know when this is. I have a sense it's early 1800's because there's nothing modern at all. There are no planes in the air. It's dead quiet in the yard around this house. There was nothing to indicate any modern appliances. For some reason, I was looking around the yard to see if there were any old tires and I see no old tires. I sort of had a sense of an old plough of some kind behind the well, but it's rusty. The kind you hook to a mule or a horse.

His description is a classic example of the kind of detail that clients report in their waking dreams. Even though he is the same gender in the dream, his physical experience of himself is clearly different. So, too, is his sense that he is living in a very different time period and geographical location.

Therapist: We have a couple of more minutes before we'll need to begin winding down for today. Notice what else it might be useful to pick up on before we adjourn until next time.

Client: I have a definite sense I'm afraid to go up this road any farther, to go over the rise. I don't know that I want to see what's on the other side of it. It's not a real hilly area, but for some reason this road peaks a little bit so that you're unable to see very far. You can only see the sky. You have to get to the top of this little hill before you can see to the other side. It's not too far up the road. Maybe a few hundred yards. The sky is still dark. It doesn't change. I feel kind of sad … Hmmm … Things are dying around there. I've walked a little bit past the house. There's an open field with a couple of large trees in the middle that are dead. They're both dead, much like that oak tree.

Therapist: There's a sense that with this drought there has come not only the death of the trees and crops but also by departure or other reasons a death of community, a death of friendship and all that is vibrant about that.

Client: Yes. It's a very empty place.

Therapist: As we come to a stopping place, I'd like you to imagine sending a message from yourself to this man that serves to bridge that emptiness if only to let him know that you share an awareness of the sadness he feels, and that you would like him to understand that there is someone who wishes to know his story, who wishes to know and understand what this sadness is about. And perhaps what preceded it that makes the sadness stand out in such contrast.

This is an invitation for him to more consciously link awareness of how he feels with the thoughts that create those feelings. Through the vehicle of compassion for the man in the dream, I am inviting him to listen to his own truth with compassion.

Client: The man that I am?

Therapist: Yes. Some people do that in a very literal way of suddenly seeing two of themselves standing there. With, on the one hand, a look of surprise of, "Where did you come from?" there is also that deep understanding within that each knows exactly where the other has come from. Sometimes with words, sometimes just with thoughts, the message is conveyed that, "I'm aware of how alone you are and the sadness of this place and this whole scene, and would like you to know I'm here to listen and to experience it with you. So that whatever this part of the journey is about, it need not be done alone."

Client: Yeah. I can see myself there on the road with him. I have my hand on his shoulder. He's much bigger than I am. I feel like I want to help him walk along the road to get over that hill, and see what's on the other side.

Therapist: Maybe we can stop at this point then for today.

This proved to be Eric's last session, as he subsequently chose not to continue in the research. At a conscious level, he offered no awareness of the parallel between the longstanding drought in his marriage and the drought that had left this scene so forlorn looking. The vacant house on the side road evoked memories of good friendships from the past, but now lay empty, with nothing there to hold him. At a symbolic level, it is easy to speculate that his own marital home had similarly come to hold nothing of value to him. At the conclusion of the session, he remained strongly hesitant to proceed over the crest of the hill, a hill that led to "a stormy sky up ahead".

Despite the expectation of rain in the dream's visual imagery, at an emotional level the suggestion is that the sadness and upset he felt over the death of his marriage still outweighed the relief he knew he would feel when he finally moved on with his life.

In my proposing that Eric insert himself into the dream, I was looking to help counter some of the isolation and loneliness that I sensed he was experiencing in his own life. Eric's image of walking up to the man and placing a hand on his shoulder held a nice mix of images:

> He's much bigger than I am. I feel like I want to help him walk along the road to get over that hill, and see what's on the other side.

Despite Eric feeling small by comparison, he believed he could offer much needed support to help the man face his fear and explore what lay ahead. Perhaps by translating the emotional experience of his current situation into a story in which the drought was a literal one, he helped himself move an important step closer to knowing he could survive the upcoming transition in his own life.

Chapter 7
The Sea Captain

Jane

Phobias are said to be irrational fears. The person has no known history that adequately accounts for the intensity of the fear that is experienced in certain situations, such as a fear of drowning or a fear of heights. If the feared situation is quite peripheral, it may have little day-to-day effect on the person's life. On the other hand, if it involves a situation that occurs frequently, a phobia can have a seriously disrupting effect. Waking dreams can often be utilized rapidly and effectively in eliminating the phobic response to the situation.

In the typical waking dream of this type, the person's death in the story is a direct link to the phobia. For example, a man with a fear of heights saw himself as a stone mason working high on a castle wall. The wind picked up, shaking the rickety ladder on which he was standing. Reluctant to climb down for fear his co-workers would ridicule him for being afraid, he clung to the ladder fearing for his life. Eventually, he chose to face his fear of being embarrassed rather than his fear of dying and he climbed down. As the waking dream progressed, the man realized he had been so scared while on the ladder that he forgot he got down safely! Like Denzel Washington's character in *Medal of Honor*, he was stuck like a videotape on pause: he kept seeing himself still on the ladder facing certain death when it collapsed. As I helped him notice what he did later that day, he was able to finish the story in his memory. He remembered that the next day he threw away the ladder and made a new one. Surveying the remainder of his life, he confirmed that he continued to work carefully when in high places, and finally died from natural causes. The client's fear of heights resolved after this waking dream.

Sometimes the phobia is linked to a chronic or episodic physical symptom. In one case, a woman, Vivian, with a fear of heights saw herself as an American Indian who fell to his death from a cliff when the ground under his feet unexpectedly gave way. Her fear had manifested as episodic left shoulder pain in situations where she felt she might lose control. Looking down on the dead body from an OBE perspective, she noticed the Indian's left shoulder had been severely dislocated in the fall. I had the two of them dialog about their respective experiences. He agreed Vivian could hold the wisdom of what he learned as he fell (i.e., to be careful when in places with uncertain footing) in her head instead of in her shoulder. Vivian's shoulder pain resolved after that session.

In another case, the woman, Jane, described it this way:

> For several years, I had an area under my shoulder blade that gave me a lot of pain. I was getting a massage once a week, chiropractic work, and bodywork. I would get relief, but it would always come back.

She had a history of anxiety attacks, which she could remember as far back as age 11, but with no known origin. Jane said she would get so scared that she feared she was going to pass out. In several different waking dreams, the pattern of fear emerged in different ways across different dream characters. As she reworked each of them, she got to the point where she no longer feared passing out, and her anxiety attacks stopped. Coincidental to this, Jane reported that her massage therapist told her, "It's like whatever was there just flew out of your body." In a follow up with her three years later, she had had no further episodes of pain in her shoulder blade, and no further anxiety attacks.

The transcript that follows involves a fear of drowning that resolved after this session. It also includes an example of how waking dreams can be used to address undesirable personality traits. Change of this type is usually slower and involves a series of waking dreams involving various manifestations of the same trait. In this waking dream, the trait dealt with the client's strong tendency to get rigid and controlling in certain kinds of social situations.

Jane is a successful corporate executive. She grew up near the ocean and remains very attached to staying near the water. She loves sailing but had had a longstanding problem with scuba diving. Her discomfort being underwater was not at the level of a true phobia, but routinely triggered a level of anxiety that was problematic for her.

Client: The ocean is such a peaceful place. I love the sea; feel like I'm rocking on it now. The salty smell, it's very peaceful. I think I'm on a ship out to sea. I'm driving the boat, a pretty big boat. I'm the captain. The waves are crashing on the front. It's fun, the bow beats down on the waves. There's works to be done. It doesn't feel like work because I love it so much. I could stay out on the ocean forever. It feels like it's dark at night. Problems. Ahoy mate, the ship's going down. I'm gagging on water. I can't breathe. Scared, palms sweating, light headed. I'm going to pass out. I'm not on the ship. I feel cold, but it will be warm in a minute.

It is unusual to move this quickly to the death of the dream character, particularly when the nature of the death was traumatic. The fact that Jane had worked with waking dreams in a number of sessions may have contributed to how the sequencing played out in this dream. Having previously experienced positive results, even with waking dreams involving a traumatic death, her mind may have "cut to the chase" on this one, moving quickly to the critical components of the dream.

Therapist: Notice that you know that.

Client: I'm going to the Light, resting now. Peaceful, I feel sleepy. The ship went down. I made a mistake. I was bullheaded about the directions. [*Here, Jane's voice tone takes on a deeper, gruffer quality.*] I'm a man, the captain of this boat. We were pulling the ropes, a frenzy, didn't have time to orchestrate it correctly. So much for those plans. Oh well, I didn't give a shit about that plan anyway. I never worried about it. I knew what I was doing, I was the captain. I never worried about that plan anyway. [*Then, noticing me more directly says,*] Who are you?

Therapist: I'm someone who helps people remember important stories and events.

Client: So why should I talk to you?

Therapist: No reason. The question is whether or not you might want to.

Client: Don't have anything else to do, might as well.

Therapist: I've been talking with another person and she was curious about what you had to deal with.

Here, I choose to stay with the dream character's experience of me as a stranger. Therapists who work with clients with a dissociative disorder will recognize the parallel here to dealing with an alter personality who emerges for the first time. Neither Jane's history nor personality testing nor behavior in therapy ever indicated she might have a dissociative disorder.

Client: You're going to tell me about Jane. [*Her voice tone switches back to her own.*] Yeah, I'm here, I get scared like that man was taking over me, like I had to come back. My heart was racing. I got scared. I don't like that man.

Her discomfort with the intensity of the dream character was a parallel to the importance she attached to being in control in her daily life. Just as a nighttime dream can involve such emotional intensity that, even upon wakening, the person still feels the emotions, Jane had excellent trance skills that enabled her to experience her dream characters so vividly.

Therapist: He has a strong sense of himself. Does he have a name?

Client: Jessup. I felt like he was taking over me. Seems like a gruff, mean man, cigarette hanging out of his mouth like a tough guy. [*Her voice tone switches back to that of the sea captain.*] Someone is shaking me. I didn't listen. I was bullheaded. I told you, I am the captain and I know it. A bunch of garbage. I'll have another puff on my cigarette. Why am I talking to you?

Therapist: [*The Captain interrupts as I make mention of the Light.*]

Client: I'm not in the Light.

Therapist: Jane discovered what you said, I made a mistake.

Client: How do you know that?

Therapist: Jane experienced it.

Client: That's a secret.

Therapist: It's a secret between the three of us now.

Client: How do I know I can trust you?

Therapist: You don't. What would help you?

Client: I don't trust many people. They try to screw you all the time. Don't trust anyone: that's the good answer. What is there not to like: I was the Captain of the ship, got my way, the ship went down.

Therapist: Did you move to the other side after that?

Client: Move to the other side of what? I'm like going along with this …

Therapist: Who is there?

Client: Jane, two guides. [*The client interjects*, "This is going to be a tough one."]

Therapist: Notice about the trust and did it work for you?

Client: I feel sad. I let people down. I wasn't very nice. I was angry, kind of a pissed off kind of guy. A lot of hard knocks. I didn't take it very well. I blamed everyone else; that made it easy. I escaped on the ship: go out to sea, get away from it all. Jane is laughing about the paper ripping [*I had just torn a piece of paper from my note pad.*] I don't know what that means. She's trying to get me to laugh, and I'm not a laughing kind of guy. Life's not very funny. Everybody always took stuff from me. I had to protect myself, so I gotta help this broad. [*The Captain did not elaborate on this seeming non sequitur.*]

Therapist: Why did it become so smart to escape to the sea?

Client: I was trying to get away from my dad—he was an alcoholic. We never lived in one place very long; always scraping for what we had. I got this job on a ship running cargo. Seemed like a good idea: be out at sea all the time, and I knew about running boats. When I was a young kid, my daddy would always be on boats. I could always be out to sea; no one could bother me living on the boats, doing my job, getting paid, a place to stay, a place to live, a place I didn't have to move all the time. When I moved I took my home was me. Seemed like a good idea. That's when I got to be sort of bull-headed, too big for my britches.

Therapist: I sense it's another thing to have people take things from you.

Client: Yeah, we a … I really don't want to talk about this.

Therapist: How about letting Jane see this? Let her move into who you were so she can experience it.

Here, I am doing a reversal of the normal screening room concept. Instead of the client having trouble with the emotional intensity of the dream, the dream character is having trouble with the intensity. By suggesting that the Captain let Jane have the experience, the Captain is able tone down the intensity for himself. Yet the effect for the client is to give her a more personal experience of being able to handle emotionally intense events.

Client: That would be easier. We lost everything when I was little. My mom got killed. It was just me and my dad. There was some kind of upheaval, everything got stolen, taken away, the house, everything. My dad being an alcoholic, what's important is my experience of it.

Therapist: What in particular was taken?

Client: My toy gun, my blanket. There was a fire.

Fire had previously been a major issue in another waking dream for this client in which the dream character had died. In that dream, the dream character had set a fire to kill a friend of hers because of jealousy over a man they both loved. However, both women had been killed in the resulting fire.

Therapist: Tell me about the fire.

Client: I was really little; I don't remember all of it. I was mad at my dad. There was warfare, we lost everything. My dad had some bad relationships. There was no one to help us. He had been drinking; he was like the town drunk. They knew it. He didn't have very many friends. Everybody looked down on me because I was his son. We didn't have anything: just mom, dad and me. Then just my dad and me. I went from school to school, I didn't even finish school. That's why I started hanging around the docks with dad, learning about boats: the lines, the winds, how to maneuver, look for storms, read the weather. I'd get on the boats and it would all go away. So peaceful on the ocean, very peaceful. My crew used to get pissed off at me, I could be an asshole, I didn't much care.

Therapist: Was it easier not to care? Was there a time when you did care?

Client: Yeah, I loved my mom and dad a lot! We were a family, before my dad got his drinking problem, or before I knew about it.

Therapist: How old were you when your mom died?

Client: Three I think. I was very sad, my mom used to protect me from my dad's anger. She would always hold me. My dad never really held me. He was even gruffer than I was, but what the hell, I could take care of myself, I learned to take care of myself.

Therapist: When did it become too expensive to care?

Client: Seven or eight I think. It hurt too much [*a particular experience*]. My dad was looking for a job. He cleaned up his act, trying to come around, take care of me; he was really going to give it a go. They wouldn't give him a break. That's when I realized you can't count on people. Count on yourself; make a way for yourself. A lot of people done worse things than me and my dad, had a lot more than we did. Seemed kind of unfair. I never really got to play in school, play kick ball, hang out with the boys. I'd see them playing in the streets laughing. I'd have to worry where the next meal was coming from, and if I could find a job, where we were going to live. Why did I have to have an alcoholic dad? Why the fuck didn't he clean up his act? The drinking just overcame him; he was distraught over mom. It's like he didn't deal with it. He couldn't deal with me, with life. What the hell did he have a kid for anyway? I wish I had some other parents. The ocean became my family, my escape, and my serenity, and as Captain I had control, so I could tell people what to do. I was sick of people telling meet where to go or what to do. I was a bratty little kid. They didn't want me around. It worked, up until it cost me my life. I feel sorry for my dad. My crew of five went down with me. I still see the waves coming over the bow; I was a dumb ass. Like the Captain of the *Titanic*, I didn't listen. I knew it all.

Therapist: The *Titanic* went down before you did?

Most of the time, the storyline in a waking dream is consistent with actual historical events. I yielded to my curiosity when this seeming non sequitur emerged.

Client: [*Jane interjects: No, an analogy. That Captain didn't listen anyway.*] [*Then in the Captain's voice again*] Jane knows that from the movie.

Therapist: And you know it from Jane?

Client: [*Ignoring my question*] Well, back then captains were like God: you didn't really challenge the Captain. That's why I liked being the Captain. When you said the orders, they did it. Some damn little whippersnapper ain't gonna talk to me. You got to be Captain 'cause you knew your stuff and the people running the boat, protecting the cargo on the ship. You gotta listen to the Captain. I got bullheaded. I was bullheaded at the wrong time. I lost my life—wasn't a great loss: no wife, kids or family, no one would miss me. Back home, who the hell cared I put the ship down. I feel kind of bad about the crew. But you know what the hell, you get on the boat—you risk that, that's part of the risk. Lots of ships during that time went down. That's what happens, take the good with the bad, know the risks. You don't have to have a bullheaded asshole Captain [*to know that.*] But I was a good sailor, I did know my shit!

Therapist: In the Light, can you let all of that be true, not just part of it?

Client: What is it about this damn light? You people make too much of this damn light. Get down to brass tacks buddy.

Therapist: Knowing you knew your shit, you were a good sailor. You got to be a captain because you knew your stuff. You knew the ocean, knew the weather, and you got bullheaded (*you* can add "asshole") and started acting like an asshole. Did you learn anything?

Client: She [*referring to Jane*] acts like a bullheaded asshole sometimes, only much different. You know, underneath this gruff I'm not that bad of a guy. I just don't like to let it out. It hurts too much.

Therapist: Maybe that's why Jane's being female, but she hung on to a lot of her masculine side, if you noticed you understand too.

Client: You're a pretty smart guy. Jane really wants to dive. She has a fear of drowning. I'll give her a gift, so she can really enjoy the water: (I'll) let her let go of that fear so she can really enjoy the water.

Hey, my guides are here, trying to soften me up. I really do have a tender heart.

While he had previously mentioned his awareness of two guides, this is the first time that there is an interaction. As I have found is always the case, the active involvement of a guide facilitates the work that is being done. Notice the dramatic shift in the tone and content of the Captain's comments that follow.

Client: Jane shows it better than I do. Jane got my take charge, bottom line attitude. Hey, by the way, she'll tell you she doesn't care about diving, but she does. She hides her fear behind her toughness. Jane needs to know that she doesn't have to be bullheaded and strong all the time. It's just a cover. Let the sweetness and the soft person out. I did that to cover up my pain. It worked for me; I had to do it at the time. Don't let it overrule her.

Don't worry about the fear of drowning. Let that fear go, it's not useful any more. Listen to people when they want to make a contribution. Probably get some good advice that might keep you from bringing the ship down. Gruffness isn't always the best way. Sometimes people aren't what you want them to be, but that's what and who they are. Don't let that get in your way. Feel like I'm talking to my little sister. The possessions of the heart are much more important than personal possessions. That's about all the softness you're getting out of me.

Therapist: What you possess in your heart and know to be true is so much more important than anything you can hold in your hand.

Client: She still has some work to do around being selfish. She gives William the sea glass freely. His radiant smile is what she takes back as her treasure: his awe and wonderment.

Jane likes to collect sea glass that washes up on the beach. In the past, she had a very difficult time giving any of it away. Recently, she had been showing it to a young boy named William and found it surprisingly easy to give him some.

Therapist: Notice if it works for you to exchange something with Jane.

Client: You're trying to get at my soft side. I'll tip my hat to her. Send her on her journey.

Therapist: What will Jane do for you?

Client: Give me a hug. She's a huggy gal; and I pat her on the back. Jane's thanking me, and I acknowledge that. It's hard for me to soften up and let people in.

Therapist: Will you fight? Will you let Jane let it in?

Client: No, I want for her happiness, but know I'll squirm. I'll honor her and squirm at the same time.

The Captain is willing to pursue what he wants—Jane's happiness—*despite* his discomfort. It is a subtle, but important, message about the way that growth normally occurs: if we are willing to tolerate being a bit squeamish like the Captain, change will occur much more quickly than if we insist on first removing all doubt and uncertainty.

This dream meshed well with another waking dream, the fire dream mentioned earlier. In the fire dream, the dream character, Susan, had offered to whisper "purple" in Jane's ear whenever Jane began acting jealous or controlling around her friends. Both Susan and the Captain addressed the notion of Jane being gentler with herself, of not needing to take things so seriously. The perceived need to see herself as always being "in control" got some permissive nudging in these and other waking dreams. For months after the "purple" dream, Jane reported that she often heard the reminder word in her head. She used this internal coaching well and worked diligently to change how she acted around her friends. The results were noticed by a number of them who commented to her on the nice shift.

We'll return to Jane in Chapter 10, where we'll take another look at some of the ways that a client's sense of the presence of spirit guides plays a healing role.

Chapter 8
Are You Sure I'm Dreaming?

Rachel

It's time for a confession. Those of you who are familiar with past-life therapy have probably recognized the many parallels that exist between waking dreams and past-life therapy. So, have you been reading about waking dreams or about past-life therapy? If I am correct, the answer is, "Yes." Let me explain.

I first became interested in the question of reincarnation in the late 1980s, but I wasn't aware of past-life therapy until I read Edith Fiore's book *You Have Been Here Before*. With my background in clinical hypnosis, Fiore's detailed descriptions provided the basis for my beginning to explore past-life therapy as a treatment tool with a few of my clients. The idea is simple enough: if hypnosis can be used to help people resolve unfinished issues stored in memory in the mind/soul, then past-life therapy can be understood as an application of this concept to events from other lifetimes. Yet as fascinating as I find the implications of reincarnation, I am a pragmatist where it comes to my use of waking dreams. My focus is on the usefulness of the dream's content as it relates to the client's presenting problem. I often use the following anecdote to summarize my reasoning on this point:

The client was a middle-aged physician who believed in reincarnation. In an earlier session, he had met a guide who had a wonderful sense of humor. After several sessions that involved imagery of the past-life kind, the client raised the question of whether there was a way to tell the difference between real past-life imagery and imagery that is just metaphorical (i.e., a waking dream). Through the client, I put this question to his guide. The client reported the following response from him:

> Yes, [*pause*] but we aren't going to tell you how to tell the difference [*pause*], because we don't want you to get distracted. [*Pause.*] And, by the way, today's imagery will be just imagery.

The remainder of the session contained a past-life-type experience that the client reported was just as vivid and just as clinically useful in addressing his presenting issues as had been his previous experiences. Since the client believed in reincarnation when he initially came for therapy, the suggestion is that the guide did not want the client to miss the therapeutic potential of the symbolic imagery by dismissing it as "not real". On the other hand, if the client's unconscious created the guide as well as the imagery, it also did a nice job of staying "meta-" to the question we had posed by reminding him to focus on the relevancy of the imagery about to be presented!

As I began to share the results of this work with some of my colleagues, I wasn't prepared for the professional backlash that occurred. One began to lecture me about the Protestant Reformation. Another thought I had joined forces with Satan and prayed for my soul. Others thought I had abandoned my scientist/academic roots in pursuit of some kind of New Age crusade.

It turns out that no serious discussion about past-life therapy can occur without confronting the question of reincarnation. In turn, it seems that no serious discussion about reincarnation can occur without confronting one's personal religious beliefs. As a profession, mental-health therapists seldom discuss theological issues with their clients, and do so even less with their colleagues. Therapists may have made good progress letting go of the illusion that mind and body function independently, but, until very recently, we have done little to let go of the illusion that mind and soul function independently. As a result, few professional organizations are yet willing to provide a forum for exploring the viability of past-life therapy as a legitimate treatment tool.

The pragmatist in me had a dilemma: I wanted a way to share my observations about this work with colleagues who were flatly opposed to the possibility of reincarnation. As a student many years before, I had learned that the best way to test an idea is to have something with which to compare it. If I wanted my colleagues to pay attention to what happens during past-life therapy, I decided I would need a different model for presenting it. What if, despite its appearances, past-life therapy isn't really about a past life? What if the imagery is purely fictitious? How could I explain why many clients (my own and those of other therapists) got better if the therapist wasn't really dealing with the consequences of events from a different lifetime? As I began to develop some tentative answers, I found myself revisiting the writings of therapists like Sigmund Freud, Carl Jung, and Fritz Perls who wrote extensively about dreams. I had additional help from two lesser-known therapists in particular, Paul Sacerdote and George Kelly, whose writings provided a critical bridge. Over a period of several years, what emerged was the model that became the basis for this book.

A number of researchers have done excellent work defining the necessary and sufficient conditions that would demonstrate that at least some people reincarnate, and collecting case studies that support the theory. For those of you who are interested, I would recommend the works of Ian Stevenson from the University of Virginia and Robert Almeder from Georgia State University (see the Bibliography). But even if one accepts the research as proof of reincarnation, it is another major step to assume that most people can easily access information from other lifetimes in past-life therapy. Given the limitations of historical records and the kind of details that are typically available during a past-life therapy session, I believe it would be impossible to research all but a very few cases. In practice, I believe that my clients probably have had a mix of sessions, some involving information from other lifetimes, and some that fit the waking dream model. When I began doing this work, I tried to be alert for clues that might distinguish between the two. As time progressed, I shifted my focus because the effectiveness of the work did not seem to have anything to do with whether the client or I thought the imagery was fictional or really from another lifetime.

There was another, even more important reason, that I gradually shifted my focus. My original fascination with the truth-or-fiction question gave way to one with more profound implications. Most, if not all of my clients, eventually encounter spirit guides, guardian angels, deceased loved ones, or other non-physical beings. Independent of the question of reincarnation, I was now confronted with how to explain these experiences. The Old and New Testaments offer numerous examples of contacts with heavenly (and demonic) beings, but few therapists would relish a meeting with the Ethics Committee armed with only a Bible! My clinical training had nothing to offer beyond openness for possibilities I had not yet considered. Like the pieces of a giant jigsaw puzzle slowly beginning to take shape, I read with excitement the writings of such authors as Gary Zukav, Michael Talbot, Ken Wilber, Gary Schwartz, Kenneth Ring, Caroline Myss, Raymond Moody, and Lewis Mehl-Madrona.

It would be easier to dismiss these encounters as simply another form of interesting fiction if their content was correlated with the religious background of each particular client. However, just as is the case with people who have an NDE, there is no such correlation. Nor is there any correlation with the client's presenting symptoms or diagnosis. The only correlation I have continued to find is that clients consistently report that these experiences are very positive. Consider this waking dream from a single woman (Rachel), an agnostic, in her twenties. In this waking dream, she saw herself as a primitive hunter:

> I was crawling in some tall grass hunting with my fellow tribesmen. My mind was not clouded with any thoughts except that I had to kill this animal in order to survive. I felt this energy with the earth as I crawled through the grass hunting my prey. There was no anger inside of me. In fact, there was not much of any emotion inside of me … My thoughts were very basic: hunger and survival. I found this incredibly enlightening … Looking at Darwinism, I can see that not only have our bodies and minds evolved, but also our emotions and feelings. It is hard to put into words what kind of experience it was to feel so simple and basic.

> I was one with the Earth. There was a harmonious feeling about the whole thing. When I died I was placed in the field to be carried away to the sun. I felt my body being lifted into the sky towards the sun. As soon as I arrived at the sun, a door appeared and I was forbidden to travel any further. The body continued to travel toward the sun, but I [*Rachel*] was not allowed to go any further. I then saw all of my lives in a circle. All of my lives are always with me; I just need to focus on one of them and it will appear. It is who I am. They all make up what I am today. I am filled with different perceptions. I see through the eyes of many people. This helps build my foundation on who I am and what I want to become.

> Being an agnostic, I had lost any kind of path or goal for my life. I was in a swirl of confusion on what the meaning of "I" was. What was the whole point of my being? Now, I have felt a deep understanding inside of myself about who I am and where I need to go.

I felt the whole Universe spinning together. I felt my past lives spinning together to form a circle. We are all in motion with the Universe; some people can't pull back and watch the cycle, and therefore try to stop the spinning and get out of sequence with the Universe. They lost harmony with the Universe. We all need to feel the spinning and not be afraid of it. I have fallen back into sequence with the Universe and have found myself along the way. Now comes the hard part; I must bring my life into sequence with the Universe.

So, are these just dreams? In the next chapter, we'll take a look at the components of a typical past-life therapy session and compare them to what happens in a typical waking dream. As you read the next chapter, it may give you a better understanding of why the question, though fascinating, pales in significance to the personal experience of developing a conscious relationship with one's spirit guide(s). I want to emphasize that the real question for me about spirit guides is not one of truth or fiction, but how these experiences can help us awaken and nurture our own spirituality and our connection with a sense of oneness with the Universe.

Chapter 9
A Typical Past-Life Experience

In Chapter 2, I gave you an overview of a typical near-death experience. Now, let's take a look at a typical past-life experience. As is the case with those who report having had an NDE, not everyone experiences all the same components of a classical past-life encounter. In particular, those that occur spontaneously are much more likely to include only some of the components listed below. Taken in sequence as they might occur in a therapy session, I find the following core characteristics:

1. The therapist helps the person move into a relaxed state of mind with the help of deep muscle relaxation, imagery, breath work, music, or some other kind of hypnotic induction.
2. The therapist makes a suggestion to move from awareness of the present time and place to another time and place. For example, in his well-known book, *Many Lives, Many Masters*, Brian Weiss instructed Catherine simply to "go back to the time from which your symptoms arise".[4] Winafred Blake Lucas offers a similarly simple suggestion, "Go back to the time when this problem first occurred."[5]
3. The person begins to see a different place, usually with a sense that it is also a different time than the present. As more details emerge in the imagery, the person develops a sense that he or she is someone else, often a different age, and frequently a different gender. Not everyone "sees" images. Some people get information as thoughts or feelings, more like an intuitive "knowing".
4. As needed, the therapist helps the person move across the lifetime of this other person. This can be done with a simple suggestion, such as, "When you're ready, you can move to the next significant scene, pausing to notice whatever seems important to bring into your awareness." This part of the experience typically takes the most time. Sometimes the person will also move to scenes from earlier in that lifetime to get a better sense of the context of what is taking place.

5. Some therapists do not deal with the death of the person from the other lifetime. Others believe that this is critical, particularly if the death was sudden or traumatic. Hazel Denning notes, "Much of the work of insight and integration from any lifetime can best be uncovered and expressed at the time that a person leaves his body in that lifetime."[6] Therapists that include this step help the person move through the death scene. The suggestions take the same form as those presented in Chapter 3. For example, "When you are ready, move to the end of your life in the lifetime you have been reviewing. Notice any circumstances that are important. When the body has taken its final breath, let me know."

6. From an out-of-body perspective following the physical death in that lifetime, the person reviews the significance of events that occurred and the conclusions or beliefs that were drawn from them. This process can be facilitated by inviting the person to meet with a spirit guide or other entity from the Light. As I discussed in Chapter 3 in the context of waking dreams, most people at this point in past-life therapy report experiences that are characteristic of an NDE. This is often a time for forgiveness and for correcting faulty assumptions or beliefs.

7. Many therapists include some kind of ritual in which the person from the other lifetime and the current person exchange a token gift to symbolize the healing that has just occurred and to strengthen the durability of the learning that has taken place.

8. The experience concludes with the client returning to a full, alert state. Like awakening from an afternoon nap, sometimes this can take several minutes or even longer.

There is nothing in these core characteristics that distinguish a past-life experience from a waking dream. There are no obvious features that help the person differentiate true memories of a past life from fictional ones in a waking dream.

Fragments of other lifetimes sometimes emerge spontaneously in unplanned ways. I have experienced this on different occasions myself while listening to music. The primary clue that such spontaneous images may really be memories from other lifetimes seems to be the emotional intensity that accompanies them. However, it is equally important to acknowledge that the emotional aftermath of current life events can also manifest at such times in this manner.

When it does, though, the imagery and associated thoughts typically have a clear linkage to the original (i.e., current life) event.

To help understand what such an experience might be like, consider the following personal example. One evening several years ago while listening to the lyrical ballad Bonny Portmore by Loreena McKennitt, I found myself suddenly experiencing imagery of the past-life type that included a profound grief reaction having learned that my husband's sailing ship had gone down in a storm off the coast of what seemed to be Ireland or Scotland. Standing on the cliffs above the town that evening, my pain was so great that I considered jumping into the ocean far below. As the imagery continued to unfold, a group of people from the town arrived and encircled me, offering silent support. Without words, we all seemed to understand that they could not force me to stay alive; that choice would always be mine. What they offered was the profound gift that I would not have to grieve alone.

Over the next several weeks, I played the song a number of times to facilitate returning to the imagery. Each time I encountered another layer of meaning. As Mary, the woman that I was in the imagery, began to wrestle with her loss, she turned for support to some of the other new widows. One of the ways in which she eventually gave new meaning and purpose to her life came in the formation of a choral group. In one of my final images, the other women and I are singing for a local audience. Embedded in the knowing glance from one of the other women came the message, "You don't have to be the whole choir; just sing your part. Trust the Director to handle the rest." The wonderful calming affect of those words has played in my ears on many occasions since then on days when my perfectionist strivings are out in full force.

Sometimes fragments from other lifetimes seem to emerge in night-time dreams. One of my clients, Karen, had a long history of nightmares that had been completely unresponsive to other therapy approaches. She regularly woke up screaming, much to the concern and distress of her husband and children. Despite her serious reservations about the question of reincarnation, she finally agreed to explore these through the use of waking dreams/past-life therapy. Over the next three sessions, Karen described the life of a young, teenage Polish girl in the early days of World War II. As she did this, her voice took on a younger quality and a heavy accent. With con-siderable distress, she described events over the next several years as the German army arrived in her town, eventually sending most of the Jews to the Warsaw ghetto. By then the Germans had already killed her father and brother. From Warsaw, the girl and her mother were sent to Auschwitz where her mother died. The girl survived, but took her own life soon after the emancipation of the camp, overwhelmed by all that she had witnessed and all that she had lost.

One of my specialties as a therapist is in working with trauma victims, but listening to her account during these three sessions was one of the most difficult things I have ever done. Had this woman in another lifetime really lived through the horrors of World War II? I don't know. Her descriptions included some details that I had certainly never encountered, such as the Ninth Fort in Poland as a place where thousands of Jews were killed during the war. Contemporary author and rabbi Yonassan Gershom has documented a number of such cases of people having memories of having lived—and died—during World War II in his book, *Beyond the Ashes: Cases of Reincarnation from the Holocaust*. What I do know is that Karen's nightmares stopped immediately after the third session. At follow up three years later, Karen had not had a reoccurrence of these nightmares.

Most forms of therapy include at least these two assumptions:

1. Past experiences (pleasant and unpleasant) shape current beliefs, attitudes, fears, wants, values, etc.
2. By going back to the time when a problem first occurred, clients can often find new solutions and resolve emotional pain.

Past-life therapy takes these two assumptions one step farther to include events from other physical lifetimes. This requires four *additional* assumptions:

3. You have a soul.
4. Your soul can incarnate many times.
5. What your soul learns from its experiences in one physical lifetime is available in other lifetimes.

6. Information from other lifetimes can be accessed consciously in various ways.

During a discussion with a colleague one day about our respective beliefs about the question of reincarnation, she commented, "God probably isn't going to change the way things work just because someone does or doesn't believe in reincarnation." When all is said and done, we either do or do not have a soul, which either does or doesn't incarnate across many different lifetimes. In no small part because of the many people with whom I have worked who have experienced terrible traumas, it is much easier for me to maintain a belief in a loving God when I work from the notion that we will all experience many, many lifetimes. It would no longer be possible for me to reject the position of existential nihilism were it not for my belief/faith that the journey of the soul is much longer and more complicated than a seemingly random roll of the dice that will determine that one's only life will end abruptly at age six in a car accident, or at age sixty as a homeless person living on the streets, or end years later with a funeral attended by thousands of mourners.

For a partially reformed perfectionist like me, my belief in reincarnation has given me some important breathing room. I no longer act as if I have to have everything just right before I die. For me, the gift of reincarnation means that this life is not a pass–fail test. I believe we are invited, indeed dared, to live each moment fully conscious and aware. We are challenged to live life fully, to experience each moment for what it is. There is no urgency to figure everything out. We have lots of time, lots of lifetimes. I think God trusts that by the time we're done, really done experiencing and learning, each soul will return to the oneness from which it came. For if God is really everywhere and everything every moment, what other final destination could our souls really have?

In the next chapter, we'll encounter some intriguing dialogue that touches on this question in the process of looking at another way in which the dream character can serve as a catalyst for personal change and growth.

Chapter 10
With a Little Help from Our Friends

Jane

Most of my clients find that they are able to access their guides more easily as they spend more time with waking dreams. Sometimes the characters from previous waking dreams re-emerge to offer their own assistance, beyond that which may have been offered during the original experience. In the waking dream presented here, Jane (from Chapter 7) got some unsolicited help from Susan, one of her earlier dream characters. Susan offered further insight and observations about Jane's progress in working on several longstanding issues. She helped focus Jane's work in two areas: the problems she continued to have with unmet expectations and her relationship with her mother. Then, later in the dream, Jane became aware of another presence:

> Wow! The light is so bright! All my guides are here and the masters, too. The love is unbelievable.

The kind of emotional support she felt for the work she was continuing to do was very reaffirming. This is typical of what other clients report with this kind of connection.

As other therapists have reported, sometimes the masters have messages for the therapist in addition to messages for the client. That proved to be the case here. As often as not, the information relayed by the client from the masters has to do with material about which the client has no knowledge.

By this time in her work, Jane had become adept at entering trance quickly. As she made the shift into a hypnotic, meditative state, I opened with a simple listing of possible areas for her to explore. As logical as the choice of topics may seem to be for a given client, I like to include a generic one at the end of the list that allows for the possibility that something else would be even more useful for the client to explore.

Therapist: A sense of humor is so important. That's why I like having spirit guides who are playful. So I would invite yours to join in the celebration today, and to join us as the room fills with light and love and laughter, and becomes an even safer place for us to use the next hour to continue to explore that which is most timely for you in this ongoing journey, this exploration, and whether it would be a good day to come back and check with Susan to see if there is more that can or might be done about her experiences as a part of your journey across time; whether the theme would be relevant of wanting someone who would take care of things and you; the theme of forgiveness; or something else that would be even more timely than those.

Client: I feel very giddy and playful today, laughing. I couldn't stop laughing earlier. [*Pause.*] I'm inviting my guides to play with us today. [*Pause.*] They're taking me to the Light first. Seems like it's been awhile since I've been there. It feels so warm on the top of my head. So relaxing. Like I could stay here. And they say, "Not yet!" [*She grins.*] Just kind of floating. I feel like I'm traveling somewhere and I don't know where I'll end up. Like I'm flying.

Therapist: I sense that it seems okay not to know the answer this time. [*She had long struggled with wanting to know the outcome of a situation before deciding if she is willing to begin.*]

Client: Yes it's okay. I was thinking, "I wonder where I'm going? Oh well. I guess I'll know when I get there." Like I'm traveling deep somewhere, deep and far. I don't know what that means. But I'm patient today! That's a miracle! I'm not going to judge anything. Write that down! [*Her guides had often teased her about the importance of her learning to be more patient.*]

Therapist: Allowing yourself the uncertainty about where you're going in no way means that you forfeit the right to return from it or deviate from it or change your mind once you do get clear about where you're going.

Client: Say the first part again.

Therapist: Not knowing the destination does not commit you to anything except the next step.

Client: I feel very sleepy, very sleepy, like I'm exhausted. Like I worked really hard, but it feels like good work. [*This sense of suddenly sleepiness correlated with significant trance deepening for her.*]

Therapist: A hard day's physical labor is often accompanied by a sense of physical fatigue that correlates with the physical labor. The same can be true emotionally.

Client: A much deserved rest. It was a rough one, whenever that means. I feel like there is a surprise somewhere. Like a little girl waiting to open her presents. Laughing, waiting for the surprise. I'm not sure where to begin.

Therapist: Has anything changed from the sense of floating?

Client: I just feel like I'm somewhere where I don't know where I am. Somebody said, [*laughing*] "Start at the beginning!" But I don't know what the beginning is.

Therapist: How about the first thought that you have?

Client: I don't know what it was. My thoughts feel empty. Like I don't have any thoughts. That's kind of weird.

Therapist: Before you rush away from that, notice what it's like to be in the place of no thought.

Client: Interesting. I don't know how I got here. It's peaceful and relaxing. It feels patient, rejuvenating, happy. It feels different. It's like someone is teaching me how to meditate. But it seems weird because I'm talking.

Therapist: Maybe it's talking that is different from thinking and analyzing. Maybe you're just verbalizing what is.

Client: That's true. I feel happy, and sleepy again.

Therapist: I would ask your guides to notice if the sleepiness is a correlation with what happens with brain wave activity during meditation. [*I elaborate on beta vs. theta brain wave activity and sleep.*]

Client: It takes a lot of patience. I'm still working on that.

Therapist: And it is hard to do that when you're physically tired.

Client: Because you fall asleep.

Therapist: And you might notice in the place where you are if there are any other sensory cues that you are aware of such as a color, or aware of any part of you that is tingling or vibrating. [*Out of body experiences that occur when awake are often accompanied by a sense that the body is vibrating as opposed to the tingling sensation which occurs when a body part "falls asleep".*]

Client: No. I thought my hands were but they aren't. I just feel like they're floating, very, very relaxed, warm. Feels very warm and safe.

Therapist: Any sense of whether the floating feels more associated with air or liquid? For example, when you're diving or floating under the water.

Client: I'm not sure. Feels like it could be either or both.

Therapist: Any sense of hearing anything?

Client: I think I can hear garbled noise. Tones and vibrations, but I can't make it out.

Therapist: Any sense of where they are in relationship to you?

Client: I think they're outside. I think maybe I'm in my Mom's tummy.

Therapist: If you want you can check with your guides to see if that is a good interpretation.

Client: Not sure. No, I think maybe it might be similar, but I'm not there. The feeling is similar; the sensation is similar. Really tired, like I could go to sleep and wake up somewhere else.

Therapist: If you would like you can move the clock forward so that that takes place.

Client: It seems like a very ancient time, further back than you and I have ever been before together. A long time ago. Maybe 500 B.C.

Notice that she did not take my suggestion to "move the clock forward" in a literal way by moving to a time in the future. Rather, she accepted the invitation to move beyond the sensations she was experiencing.

Therapist: They wouldn't have known that, but if the reference is helpful.

Client: Very long ago, but there is something important for me there. I don't know what it is. Where something started, where it all started. Like the very beginning; where a connection for me started. Some stone ... [*This gives more meaning to the earlier comment she heard in her head to "Start at the beginning!"*]

Therapist: As much as you can, remember to be careful to simply observe and report rather than to explain and make sense.

Client: It has something to do with stone, or a stone room, a cave. Like I have a rock, pounding on a rock. There are not many people, a small group—I think that's what we call ourselves—a village. Kind of fuzzy. Trying to remember like its way deep in my memory.

Therapist: [*I offer a suggestion for trance deepening.*]

Client: I don't know why the word "deep" keeps coming up. Deep in my memory, deep in my psyche. Not necessarily anything bad or scary, just a long time ago.

Therapist: What if you send a message to this person back in 500 B.C. that you would like to listen to or see this person's story.

Client: It has something to do with some teaching. Somebody teaching.

Therapist: Focus on a different way of knowing, perhaps on visuals instead of linguistics.

Client: Seems like some writings in a cave. A fire that we sit around. It doesn't seem like there are any women there, just some men. Kind of like cave men. I think I'm the leader talking to them.

Therapist: Are you aware of your gender?

Client: I must be a man.

Therapist: Why?

Client: Because there are no women there. It seems like [*she laughs*] like Fred Flintstone-ish. But I think I have long hair, some cloths on [*she points to her waist and lower torso*]. Something about a plan.

Therapist: Notice the mood of those around you in the room.

Client: I don't think that's important. I don't know why we're here.

Therapist: Is it okay to know?

Client: Yes.

Therapist: Convey that thought, that with this context you'd like to get some additional awareness and understanding about what is important, either in this place or as a prelude to something which comes later.

Client: I think it has something to do with you. I don't know what though. I can't figure it out. It seems like so many years ago. How can that be possible?

Therapist: Nature has been working on the Grand Canyon for about one million years. It's still in the same place. The water has carved its way down.

Client: I feel like someone is saying that I'm so damn stubborn. Why would someone say that! [*Exasperated.*] I try hard. I don't know what I'm being stubborn about.

Therapist: Stubborn is a perception of the viewer. The one who is perceived as stubborn tends to label herself as persevering.

Client: [*There is a distinct voice tone change here that is consistent with that of Susan.*] Well I guess I'll just have to handle this for her since she can't on her own.

Therapist: Welcome.

Client: That girl is so stubborn. It is just amazing to me. She's got a damn hard head. I swear I'd hit her over the head if I could. Sometimes I just laugh at her.

Therapist: That is like earlier in today's session when she was laughing at something that someone else had said about her.

Client: Poor girl, she tries so hard. She lets that damn logical side get in the way.

Therapist: Is there another word that you could give her for "stubborn" that she may resonate to in a better way?

Client: Fixed, controlling, domineering. Shall I go on? [*Laughing.*]

Therapist: You wanted a chance to hit her over the head! You might want to check with her and see if she recognizes any of them. Fixed?

Client: She's squirming a little bit. She doesn't always recognize them. "Fixed" means not being flexible, not going with the flow, not listening to her damn heart.

Therapist: [*I comment about an incident in the session the day before when the client had denied something and then two minutes later acknowledged that she had done so.*]

Client: She is practicing. It's a connection with you. And she just sits there saying, "That's not right. That's not how I pictured it. That's not what I thought it was."

Therapist: At the risk of saying something that doesn't need to be said, is that like when someone decides what form the solution has to look like and then rules out every other solution because it doesn't look like what they said it had to look like?

Client: Yes.

Therapist: Am I in the cave there, too?

Client: Yes.

Therapist: Do you want to point me out to her?

Client: She doesn't use her instincts, her intuition enough. Not near enough and I don't know how to help with that.

Therapist: Is there anything about the imagery she is looking at in the cave that has anything to do with her turning away from using and honoring intuition?

Client: Just logically, it didn't make sense to her. So she wasn't going to speak it.

Therapist: How about the man in the cave? Is there anything that happened to him in that life that led him to turn away from relying on his intuition? [*In keeping with Jane's comment about the Flintstone quality to the scene, I'll call the man Barney.*]

Client: That's why they call you the "Doc!" [*Grins.*] He didn't want to listen to what anybody was telling him. No, he listened to what people were telling him. It's both, what people were telling him and listening to himself. I see myself hitting her on her hands. [*Laughs.*] I wonder how she got so damn hard-headed. Actually, I know how she got that way. She hasn't discovered that yet. [*I resisted the temptation to get off on a tangent pursuing the implication.*]

Therapist: What else is there about her life as that man in the cave that would be relevant here, that by re-experiencing it she could connect with the importance of listening both with one's ears and one's intuition?

Client: Bullheadedness.

Therapist: Were there consequences to [*Barney's*] bullheadedness?

Client: I don't know that that's important. It's not. As a man in that lifetime he did not show his feelings. Everything was always business. His way or no way. The council would try to tell him but he would not listen, period, because he knew all the answers. He thought he had all the answers. And he didn't, and he needed their help but he just wouldn't listen. You were on the council with him, tried to help him and teach him, but he wouldn't listen to you either. But she listens to you now though. He ruled with a hard, heavy hand. Not very feeling. He hurt some people on the council.

Therapist: As you are telling me this I hope she is having an opportunity to experience that.

Client: [*Sigh.*] You know that girl. She got the message. The man shut people out. Didn't let them in.

Therapist: Is it important to understand how he came to that decision to shut people out?

Client: No. He was just a very cold, hard nosed ruler of the council. My time is so short today. I can't stay much longer, and I really, really wanted to ask a question about forgiveness.

Therapist: Do you want to address that before you go?

Client: She has begun to open that door of forgiveness, but she's got to kick it open a little further. It is just a crack right now. She did some good cleanup with her dad. She's got to work on her mom now. She's not learning what she can from that relationship, blocked by her lack of ability to forgive and to love unconditionally. She only loves her mom conditionally. And she believes the conditions have not been "worthy" of her love.

Therapist: She knows that her guides love her despite the "conditions"?

Client: All-in-all she can be a real bitch sometimes!

Therapist: [*Smiling.*] I wonder if that's why she commented that her coming home party has something to do with that? [*She had earlier told me that her friends were naming the party, "The bitch is back."*] And you know what? I think they would love her even if she wasn't a bitch. I think she needs to know that though.

Client: Yes, I think she does.

Therapist: That she won't give up her power if she gives up being a bitch.

Client: She doesn't see it.

Therapist: And just in case she needs to hear it, I forgive her for not listening to me back there in the cave.

Client: She listens very deeply and very intensely to you now … Back to this thing with her mom. It's not about right and wrong, but she wants to put it in the right and wrong category. It's about unconditional love and being able to open her heart and arms [*in a figurative way*] standing in the face of being pissed off. It's just like her friend: staying connected even when you're in the trigger. And that's what it is for her. Because believe me: her mom can trigger her!

Therapist: And what if the gun was loaded with blanks? Or better yet, what if the gun simply had an empty cartridge? You could pull the trigger all you want and nothing would fire.

Client: She's always got the bullets coming at her. Or sees them as bullets.

Therapist: If each bullet exploded into a flower blossom or fireworks, or transformed into a rainbow of color before it got to her ...

Client: That would help. See, in the place where she is right now, she can't help her mom. Her mom needs some spiritual growth. She is struggling in this lifetime with her development and Jane could help her. But the place that Jane is in does not lend itself to help her. Her mom can not listen to her. And it's not her mom's fault. Jane speaks and her voice has daggers in it.

Therapist: So her mom uses bullets and Jane uses daggers?

Client: Right. And they're just sparring with each other, and that's not good. You and Jane work on her mama before she goes back to [*her home state*].

Therapist: Okay.

Client: That's going to be a good help for her: [*It will*] free up some space when she can open up that door to forgiveness.

Therapist: To the extent that there is anything left over from your life, Susan, that has a parallel here, just in case this issue fits in some way on your end, you, too, can help Jane by role modeling what's involved in giving and getting forgiveness.

Client: I have forgiven, totally. I have opened up my heart. I've let Barney back into the circle with no problem, and I'm moving toward the Light. You know I'm not in the place on hold anymore.

Susan is referring to a waking dream in which she was the main character. In that dream, Susan had set a fire to kill a friend of hers because of jealousy (see Chapter 7). However, both women had been killed in the resulting fire. In the out-of-body experience after Susan's death in the dream, she had found herself in a much darker place than most of my clients' experience, a kind of "holding place". She did not have the experience of being in the Light following her death in that lifetime. Her description was much more in keeping with the religious concept of "limbo".

Therapist: I don't know if Jane knew that.

Client: She didn't. I'm in a much better spot. She's freed me up, and I still have some work to do.

Therapist: Can you accept forgiveness now?

Client: Yes I can. Yes I can. I've been in the Light. It's been so wonderful. I've been giddy, too, laughing with Jane today. Celebrating her move. That was the secret I couldn't tell.

Here, Susan seems to be alluding to the idea that she is no longer in "limbo". Parallel to the work that Jane has been doing, Susan seems to have been hard at work on her own issues.

Therapist: Did you know about the move?

Client: Yes. And she was being hard headed about it! And while we're on the subject, she needs to pick up the damn phone and call that man about the land. Quit pussy-footing around. Sometimes I'm amazed that she is so successful! If her destiny has always been to be back in [*her hometown*], she has some work to do there. Lots of connections for her there. She's only just begun. [*Smiling.*] I can't tell you any more than that.

Therapist: And if she has been working on it for 2500 years, then I would say she has more than just begun, and yet in some ways she's only just begun. [*Like the client in the next chapter, Jane also believes in reincarnation.*]

Client: Yes, it is both. She's only just begun in this incarnation.

Therapist: And if she's been working on things for 2500 years, then there is no hurry that she finishes things in this lifetime.

Client: [*Laughing.*]

Therapist: So maybe she can relax a little bit, and like you, she can enjoy the giddiness of those moments of success when the pieces do come together; when serendipity and synchronicity are recognized and *being* feels so good.

Client: I don't want her to think she's not recognized for all her efforts, because she is. I'm just trying to push her a little more, to open up a little more to recognize the things she still has left to work on.

Therapist: I will ask this to check my assumption, that you are pushing her more because you know she's capable.

Client: Oh, very capable. And she has lots of recognition and self-awareness. There are just some areas where she's got blind spots, like we all do. And it's hard for her sometimes to accept them.

Therapist: My quote of the week has been attributed to Frank Zappa who is quoted as having said, "Reality is what it is, not what we wish it to be." And I hear a message for Jane that when reality is what it is, that before she says it's not what she thought it should be, would be, ought to be, could be, or must be, that she simply name it for what it is.

Client: And you know, that darn girl, she knows about all those shoulds and oughts and all that. She just goes in the inner turmoil, swirling around up there in that brain of hers. I just say, "Spit it out!"

Therapist: So let's put her back in the cave for moment.

Client: Wait a minute. I just say, "Spit it out, bitch! Go ahead."

Therapist: Let's put her back in the cave for minute.

Client: Okay.

Therapist: In the circle. The council is around her talking to her, and she/he sees me in that life there in the council. And I would like to invite Jane to just acknowledge that. Simultaneously acknowledging with the other hand the surprise or disbelief or mismatch between expectations and what is, which is a way of recognizing that expectations were different than what is when there is surprise or disbelief.

Client: Yes, you know what? That is a very valid point you bring up, because she struggles with managing expectations. That is a struggle for her. Put that on your list.

Therapist: Okay. We can't be surprised or disappointed or upset or confused, except that we thought ahead and developed an expectation about what would happen at that point in time. She had an expectation about what it would look like in a life in which she and I were together.

Client: Right. And I think this is important to note, how little the expectation can be to screw things up. Her expectation was just not that it would be 500 B.C. in a cave. Nothing more than that. But it was not. That's all. And that's enough. [*Much has been written about the power of positive expectations. This is a lovely message about the negative power (consequences) that expectations can also carry.*]

Therapist: Right.

Client: It only has to be so little.

Therapist: No trouble. [As an aside regarding her double entendre here about my tendency to talk too much:] Getting me to shut up in a group is tough. That's why I work solo.

Client: [*Laughing.*] And I was just going to say, I struggle with that running of the mouth like you do!

Therapist: So in the cave I invite Jane to notice what is, and to notice that her expectation was different from what is. To simultaneously be aware of both. That expectation is the result of thought, of evaluation, of analysis. And then, the good manager/listener pays attention to see if what happens matches expectations. If not, notice that it doesn't, and take full advantage of both the match and the mismatch to develop the next set of expectations.

Client: And she's not even sure how to manage the thoughts when they come, the thoughts that are expectations.

Therapist: What if we call them "hypotheses" instead of "expectations"?

Client: You mean as a way to help her?

Therapist: Yes. That if she generated a set of "hypotheses" about what might be.

Client: I think that could work.

Therapist: And then like the scientist, observe what happens to notice what it tells her about her hypotheses.

Client: Like when you have her question things sometimes. Asking questions rather than expecting just an answer.

Therapist: Or when we make a list like we did today at the beginning of five possible topics. We always include a sixth one which is,

"Or whatever else might be even more important than these." That way, we're never wrong, because we always include in the list a recognition that no matter how complete our list, we're open to the possibility that because of things we don't already know about, something else might indeed make even more sense. Thus the sixth hypothesis. Then, instead of expectations that function as limiting, as fixed, as a set within which the answer has to fit, her hypotheses become an open-ended set of possibilities which always includes the extra one at the end: "And anything else I haven't already thought of."

Client: By the way, you notice I'm getting to stay longer?

Therapist: Yes.

Client: The guides are letting me because of the different place I've moved to.

Here, Susan seems to be confirming what she implied a few minutes earlier: that she is no longer in the dark place of limbo that she was following her physical death. With the help of her guides, she seems to have done some needed growth/healing work that has enabled her to move to a different place.

Therapist: I like cause and effect.

Client: Yes, I thought you'd enjoy that.

Therapist: I don't know that it's important for Jane so much as it is a curiosity for me of what it is about the place where you were that put constraints on how long you could stay?

Client: It has to do with cause and effect in that a holding place is a place for kind of like repenting, and having to rebuild from where you began. And so the times are limited. Having said that I do have to go today.

Therapist: Congratulations for what it means that you were able to stay longer.

Client: Thank you. It means a progression and a growth for me. And thanks for your work also because it all comes together in the universe as you know.

Therapist: Yes.

Client: And I hope you can help Jane [*sigh*] not be so stubborn!

Therapist: [*Laughing.*] I enjoy the challenge.

Client: And she can be challenging! I've enjoyed our time together today.

Therapist: In case we don't meet again for whatever reasons, since it all ultimately is part of one anyway, I note that the spirit of your thoughts and energy and love for Jane's manifestation of the soul from which I sense you both derive will certainly be present.

Client: Always. They're calling me back now. I have to go home as much as I'd like to stay.

I want to step out of the waking dream for a moment to comment on the meta-level meaning. Once again we get the sense that "Susan" has traveled across some dimension of space and time in order to participate in this session. In considering alternative explanations, I would note, again, that nothing in Jane's history ever raised the possibility for me that she might have developed other personalities in the past as a response to trauma. If, as a clinician, you've never had the experience of carrying on a conversation like the one taking place here, you may find yourself confronted with a version of Jane's dilemma regarding pre-existing expectations or beliefs: How do we explain what has been taking place in this session with regards to "Susan", whose voice tone and style are distinctly different from Jane's? Who or what is "Susan"? While I find these questions extremely stimulating, as a pragmatist I invite you to focus for the moment on the clinical meaning for Jane of what just took place. For several months preceding this session, "Susan" has been functioning in the manner of an operant conditioning cue, calling to Jane's attention social situations where Jane was acting jealous, possessive, etc. The positive changes in Jane's behavior had been noted by a number of her colleagues and friends. Now, in this session, "Susan" has proffered several important pieces of clinically useful information:

• Through the vehicle of this waking dream in which Jane has perceived me as another character in the dream, "Susan" has succinctly observed that Jane struggles with situations where reality doesn't match her expectations, and that even a small mismatch can result in Jane becoming stuck. This leads to a reframe to call them "hypotheses" rather than "expectations".

- "Susan" functions to encourage Jane to stop remaining silent when she encounters a mismatch. "Susan" steps forward to tell me about this when Jane was unwilling to speak about either her sense that I was one of the council members, or that she had expected I would eventually show up in one of her waking dreams—just not like this. Note how "Susan's" delivery comes from a place of deep caring while allowing a simultaneous expression of exasperation that includes a heavy dose of humor. If the printed version of this doesn't convey it clearly, I will ask you to trust me that when "Susan" spoke, her voice tone conveyed all of this quite well.

- "Susan" informs me that Jane has important work to do regarding her relationship with her mother, parallel to previous work she had already done regarding her relationship with her mother.

- "Susan" speaks to the power and importance of forgiveness and redemption as change agents.

- "Susan" role models for Jane in a playful way that it is possible to explicitly acknowledge another person's shortcoming (my tendency to get long-winded at times) in a way that maintains balance and mutual respect (she acknowledged her own tendency).

Whoever or whatever "Susan" really was, I found her to be a very useful co-therapist whose contributions to Jane's therapy were consistently relevant and constructive.

Returning to the closing moments of the session:

Therapist: Have a good trip.

Client: [*Jane returns.*]

Therapist: We have a couple minutes left in case you want to add anything.

Client: I don't have that feeling anymore, this change when she would go. Another scary one? I didn't have it. Wow! The light is so bright! All my guides are here and the masters too. The love is unbelievable.

114

Therapist: You just said something I'm curious about if it can be elaborated on: that both your guides and masters are here. Is there a way to explain the difference between them?

Client: Yes, the masters are of a higher plane. My guides are of a lower plane spiritually and my masters are of a higher plane. We all have guides and masters. Sometimes they work separately and sometimes they work together. The masters teach the guides. The guides are more available than the masters.

Therapist: That would make sense, just like in a company with supervisors.

Client: The masters oversee more of the bigger universal issues, but they are tied to me also. And the love is incredible! They say, "Sometimes Susan has a sharp tongue, but a truthful one," and that I have been working hard on my growth. Not hard, diligently. Big difference.

Therapist: Good choice of words.

Client: Sometimes because growth is uncomfortable at times I label it as hard. But it's really not hard. Diligent or committed are better words. My masters say that they want to tell you that you do good work, too, and to keep it up, and that your path is going to be changing some, too. This is your real calling this work, and it's beginning to move more in this direction. They acknowledge the paper you wrote as a step 7 and that there is some other work that you're thinking of doing or doing in that direction. Moving this type of therapy to the forefront. Having it be a different model of viewing, not so threatening.

Therapist: [*I comment on the timing of their observations as they relate to other professional events that were taking place that month. Jane was not previously aware of those professional events.*]

Client: It's time, and you know what the answer is! They say its time for you to grow now. Just to step out there, and they'll provide openings for you, a path, and you know that. You just haven't been willing to take the step. It's a different time now than it was (when you got started). And don't get stuck thinking about that time. The universe has shifted, and this type of therapy is shifting. Universally, they are creating the space too, but the Universe is also, and the timing is right now for you.

115

> **Therapist:** Enjoy a few closing minutes with them, asking for any final messages that fit.

Here, we have seen another example of how a dream character can interject herself in a different waking dream to help the client make additional progress on major personality issues. In a variation of how Dorothy got help from Claire, Jane got help from Susan. This time, however, the help was offered without the client going through the death of the current dream character. While we can speculate on the meaning for the client of finding me in this story, the primary message seems to have been this: even a minor mismatch between expectations and reality can result in a person getting stuck if she is unwilling to allow reality to be different from her expectations.

Susan functioned as a compassionate observer whose advice could be heard easily by the client without "resistance" as it came from within rather than from the therapist. Clients rarely, if ever, reject the suggestions they get from the characters in waking dreams. From my vantage point as the therapist, I cannot remember a time when I have been uncomfortable with the advice being given to a client in this fashion. In this way, I enjoy using both the dream characters and the client's guides as co-therapists. Occasionally, when I query the guides about the timing of something for the client to consider, they have recommended postponing it until another piece of work is completed. On other occasions, they have cautioned me to keep the client focused on the issue at hand. I find it striking that clients relay these messages from their guides with no apparent hesitation. I suspect their willingness to do so is a function of their knowing (not just hoping) that the guides have the client's best interests at heart.

Jane concluded the bulk of her work with me several years ago. The following year, she moved out of state but was able to come back for two brief periods to do some additional work. Since then she has sent me an occasional e-mail to let me know how things are going for her. In one, she wrote a more extensive summary of the changes she has seen in her life since she began therapy:

> I thought in therapy I was going to address the issues I had with the inability to have successful love relationships. I had been through a

divorce one year earlier. I was in a new relationship and the same patterns were emerging. So, on that day, I began an incredible journey.

What I didn't know was the degree to which healing could occur, the depth at which healing could occur, and the depth at which my spirituality and understanding of myself, my family, and my life learning's would be expanded. I had no sense of how life altering this journey would be.

We started out addressing the issues that I had around male love relationships ... What ended up happening was the ability for me to have a conversation with my father that I had yearned to have for over 20 years. This healed some deep wounds that allowed my heart to open up, which gave room for my soul mate to finally come into my life. I now have the relationship I have always dreamed of having.

... I have saved what I say is the best for last: the spiritual growth and universal understanding I experienced. I remember the first time my guides were there, I told Dr. Schenk, "Be quiet, someone is talking to me." I was giddy, and very light hearted. I truly understood in that moment what "laying on hands" means; I felt like they were all around me with their hands on me, (and they were). The wisdom and love I felt, the deep connection to myself and the world is unexplainable. Your guides are here all the time, nudging you, loving, guiding you. I began to receive messages from them for myself and for other people. I began to feel the synchronicity of life. There are no coincidences; everything happens for a reason. We are given free will and the different choices we make will put different learnings in front of us. Your guide will always want to walk with you on the path that is for your highest good and best spiritual growth. I am still on the path, walking with them by my side.

Chapter 11
A Lesson about Love

Jenny

Just as my clients come with diverse personal histories, they also come with diverse spiritual perspectives. As a part of my intake, I inquire about their religious and spiritual beliefs. Some have a traditional view of heaven and hell as destinations after physical death. A few believe that this is all there is; that there is nothing following death. In recent years, an increasing number of my clients have voiced a belief that their souls reincarnate in many lifetimes. This upsurge has been paralleled by a spate of books, movies, and TV shows that include various permutations of this theme.

Sometimes a waking dream seems to slam right into a thorny religious/spiritual issue. Such was the case with Jenny, a single woman in her late forties with a long history of significant intestinal problems. In the years since I had first seen her, she had continued to make good progress with her physical health. Now she had come back to therapy to work on a relationship with a man she had begun to date. His own history where relationships were concerned had left him understandably skittish about the prospects. Jenny was finding dating to be hard work, and was tempted to give up on this new relationship. In the excerpt that follows, the dream character chose to commit suicide following the death of someone whom she loved dearly. The dream character went on to describe some unanticipated consequences that help demonstrate the significant overlap between psychotherapy and spirituality.

In this waking dream and the excerpts from two subsequent sessions, Jenny got help from the dream characters and her guides on understanding the differences between attachment and love, and the importance of achieving a healthy balance between love directed at others and love that is given back to self.

Hypnosis came easily for Jenny as she had considerable experience with meditation. We began this session by inviting the presence of a dream character, Angelica, from an earlier waking dream. In that earlier waking dream Jenny, had remarked:

> She [*Angelica*] wants to show me that human love, though sometimes short-lived, is a tremendous blessing. It doesn't matter how long it lasts, really. It just matters that it exists, human love. Human love of receiving and giving. It's like an instant when I see this shimmering of the tree or the leaves—the God that exists within it. The one instant and then the next time I may not notice when I walk by the same tree, but the instant, while short-lived, has great impact on the one who experiences it. The impact is very recognizable in the moment, and the subtle effect is less recognizable though extraordinarily valuable, too.

When she gave the example of the shimmering of the tree, I was reminded of the wonderful scene in John Travolta's movie, *Phenomenon*, in which he seems to have exactly this kind of experience while gazing at a grove of trees outside his home.

As Jenny put herself in a deep meditative state, I reminded her of Angelica's closing words in the earlier session inviting Jenny "to be and have faith". The following waking dream emerged a moment later:

> **Client:** Well, it's … what is it? It seems I was a little girl in a pretty dress, a happy little girl in a pretty dress. Yup. And a brother that I looked up to and admired and loved. Two parents were there. A seemingly happy situation. It was a happy situation. It wasn't that long ago. It seems very American but I'm not sure. It seems very familiar. The little boy was very much of a caregiver of sorts in terms of caring for the little girl. He would hold her hand across the street; have a watchful eye and a kind heart.
>
> The two growing older, teenagers, continue to be very fond, very affectionate, with a great, great love for one another. Now it's time for the little boy to go away. The little boy is a teenager. I, as the little girl, am deeply saddened. We write letters. Sort of a rosy picture, like a storybook.
>
> The brother seems to have been killed somehow.
>
> **Therapist:** Notice if it is important to know how.

Client: It was an accident with a horse on a field. It was time for him to go. The sister is inconsolable. [*Jenny continued to describe what she saw in a mix of first- and third-person perspectives.*] Their relationship was certainly one of brother and sister, but with a deeper love than most, a very strong emotional connection. So when he died I or she—I don't know whether to speak in "I" or "she"?

Therapist: Notice that you have been staying third person.

Client: First person is harder here. Ugghhh. I start to feel bad [*in the first-person experience*]. My stomach is hurting now.

When someone describes the dream from a third-person perspective, it is often because it helps tone down the emotional intensity. When the client is willing, I encourage him or her to shift to a first-person perspective to enhance the impact of the experience.

Therapist: It may be important, then, that you do this in the first person.

Client: I don't want to live any more. I just don't see the point. I don't care about anybody at all. I don't want to go on. I don't understand. I don't even care to understand. It seems that suicide is the best option. It's just too hard to think about how, how would that happen. I don't know, but that's certainly the best option. Oohhh! Wooooooooohhhhhh! My stomach is tight. I think that a knife would be useful. Mmmmmmmm. So, [*sighs*] what will I do with a knife? I have an image or a feeling that stabbing myself in the heart, Uugggghhhh. [*Long pause.*] Can I do this? Can I do this? [*Sighs.*]

Therapist: Know that if you'd like, you can fast forward to see the results of whatever your final decision is.

I had previously taught her the screening-room technique that enables clients to treat the dream imagery as they would a videotape. In their imagination, they can use a remote control device to freeze the action, fast forward over a difficult section, mute the volume, or rewind to a previous scene. This technique is very helpful when dealing with emotionally intense imagery.

Client: Okay. [*Pause.*] It was stabbing to the heart. Now I am in the place of no more body. However, this place post-stabbing/suicide is not full of light or painlessness.

121

Therapist: Can you still see the body?

Client: Yes, I can.

Therapist: Before you leave where the body is, would you notice whatever there may be which is important about the physical injuries.

Client: There is so much blood. Mmmmmm. There is so much pain to the parents. Oh it hurts to have hurt the parents! There is a great debt to pay for this action. My stomach still hurts.

Therapist: Describe the debt.

Client: [*Sighs.*] The act of selfish suicide and the pain it caused creates great karmic debt for future lifetimes. It is not the will of God that one should be so self-absorbed and unconcerned with how actions hurt others. The debt [*moans*] is long lasting and will manifest in the future in different ways. One way is with great loneliness. Another is with being abandoned by others as I was. Another is with disappointments, expectations. Another is with the experience of spending a lot of time alone with longing. There is a Universal law about suicide. There is a lesson to be learned, many lessons to be learned. A big lesson is manifesting in this [*Jenny's*] lifetime with my unconscious belief that love is too hard. So it is important [*sigh*] to make or let or allow or learn in this life that love can work. It will be of utmost importance to learn that lesson. It is the biggest lesson. So, yeah, I don't know how to learn that lesson.

Over the course of time, a number of my clients have reported waking dreams in which they used suicide as the solution to a difficult situation. Independent of the client's prior personal beliefs, the consequences of the suicide in the dream imagery showed striking similarities. The normal sense of peace and tranquility following death from any other cause was conspicuously absent. In its place were various descriptions of a setting that had the emotional equivalent of being in limbo. Before being able to move from this place into the Light, the person had to first grapple with the larger implications and consequences involved in a death by suicide. As was the case with Jenny, many clients have reported an understanding that this learning would be played out over several *lifetimes.* I would note, however, that in each case the suicide involved a person who was physically healthy. Therefore, I would not extrapolate these observations to situations involving someone who is in the final stages of a fatal illness.

Therapist: Would you invite the brother to join you and notice if it is important to understand why it was his time to go?

Client: Oh, it was his time to go. He experienced unconditional love and he gave generously of himself. He had to help me release attachment—attachment—strong attachment. He had done his job. While he was there on the other side the soul still had darkness at first.

Therapist: Whose soul?

Client: My soul after the suicide had darkness. His soul was great white light. [*Sigh.*] So the connection was not continued. Hmmm. The soul, the person who commits suicide pays a debt for a long time after and does not stay without a body for very long. There is darkness between the lifetimes.

Therapist: Were you given any assistance between lifetimes?

Client: Yes. What was it? Can't quite see what it was. Certainly a push into the next lifetime. That was some of the assistance.

Therapist: Your push or their push?

Client: Their push. My stomach-ache is gone.

Therapist: Would you meet with who you were when she attempted to end her pain in the way that she chose, and notice the parallels between her stomach pain and the form of the physical symptoms you have had in this lifetime (and any other parallels that exist)? Is it possible now having heard her story and felt her pain that you can honor the wisdom and lessons you have learned without holding it in the physical body in the same way that she did?

Client: It seems that the majority of my abdominal pain and suffering in this life has since passed, for the most part. There could be some remaining residual that is not ready to depart. However, certainly the majority has passed. There is some pain in the heart from having stabbed the heart and the manifestation in this lifetime is a fear of pain in the heart. Therefore it takes time and trials and errors. [*She interjects: "Are there errors? Maybe so."*] To test and find out

> with little baby steps if the pain is going to be felt. So that fear of heart ache is very real, though not conscious.
>
> **Therapist:** Would you please take some time to create a healing ritual that honors the emotional pain she felt in her heart chakra before her death, and acknowledges the correlation of that stabbing pain from her physical act of stabbing the heart as a recognition of how intense her emotional heart pain was, and inviting the guides to join you in a ceremony aimed at bringing healing light energy to that space, the emotional heart and removing the physical knife as someone certainly did when he or she found her body.

This healing ritual can be modified to handle a wide variety of situations. At its core are a few basic components: an acknowledgment of a prior emotional pain, a recognition of how it was paralleled with physical symptoms or illness, and permission to allow full healing to occur at all levels. This requires (1) addressing the relevant thoughts and beliefs about the event, (2) the resulting feelings, and (3) any way in which the physical body mirrored or was involved in those events.

> **Therapist:** And perhaps as silversmiths will do, melting that which the knife was made of into a different shape. Perhaps a heart shape or some other shape.
>
> **Client:** The shape is one of a heart that says "love yourself". I see that one of the mistakes I made as that girl was to love my brother as myself instead of loving myself as well. It was outer directed, completely outer directed which is where the attachment comes in. So loving myself. Yup.

Jenny regularly cross-checked things she said by noticing how she *felt* about what she had just said. When there was a clear match, she would typically utter, "Yup."

> **Therapist:** Can the energetic form of that heart be given to you as a gift to go into your own heart space, as a basis for healing and fuller awareness?
>
> **Client:** Yes. It's being given as a gift.
>
> **Therapist:** Notice whether or not there are any attachments.
>
> **Client:** No there are not any attachments.

Therapist: You might thank her for that. She seems to have learned her lesson about attachments.

Client: Okay. [*Long pause.*] She is learning that attachments can cause pain and disappointment. It is a great lesson to learn how to love without attachment, and one not completely learned yet.

Therapist: Notice if you can love being a work in progress.

A number of clients, especially those who are rather perfectionistic, experience an immediate, strong affective response/shift when I have them say aloud the following sentence: "I give myself permission to be a work in progress."

Client: Yes, absolutely. Yes, yes, yes. [*Long pause.*] The work in progress continues with a great deal of accomplishment having been made. Twenty years ago when the teaching about attachment arose, there was no understanding. It was very confusing. Confusion between attachment and love. I didn't know the difference. I'm now seeing and learning and experiencing the differences.

Therapist: Are you aware of the presence of your guides?

Client: Yes.

Therapist: [*We have a brief discussion about an additional resource person with whom she is working.*] I ask, then, that your guides and hers [*those working with the resource person*] work with you both to help that work be as useful and constructive as possible.

Client: Yes.

Therapist: Anything else before we close?

Client: No. Gratitude. Just gratitude.

It is an interesting concept, the idea of being a work in progress instead of expecting ourselves to be "finished" at some point in our lives. The world around us offers many parallels that can influence our personal expectations in subtle ways. My younger son and I enjoy watching new homes being constructed. As works in progress, it is fascinating to see each home taking shape. Though not yet a teenager at that point, my son had already developed a good eye for visualizing the floor plan once the stud walls were in place. But what he enjoys most is walking through a model home in a new subdivision. This kind of home is complete; it is no longer a work in progress. The carpets are spotless, there is no chipped paint on the molding, the windows are clean.

Many of my clients seem to have a subtle belief that their own life can, and should, ultimately reach this state of completion. A new car can be assembled in a matter of weeks. A new house can be constructed in a few months. Man set foot on the moon less than 10 years after President Kennedy's famous speech that defined that goal. So perhaps it is not surprising if, at midlife, people reflect on their lives and wince to discover that they are still very much works in progress.

If, then, our entire lives can be seen as an ongoing work in progress, negotiating that process can be easier with the help of a seasoned coach or mentor. When faced with an unfamiliar or difficult situation, it is nice to have someone to turn to for advice and support. As a therapist, I enjoy the opportunity to serve in this capacity for my clients. Yet even more than this, I enjoy helping my clients develop (or strengthen) a conscious connection with their own spirit guides. No appointment is necessary; there are no authorizations needed nor insurance forms to complete; they are available at any hour of the day or night.

A brief tangent is in order here. When I direct a question to a guide, clients usually "hear" the answer in their heads and relay it to me. Some clients, however, seem to allow the guide to speak through them. When this occurs, the client is always referred to in the third person. There is often a shift in voice tone. For some there is a shift in the kind of vocabulary and sentence structure that is used. Such shifts are consistent with the phenomena of full trance channeling in which a person is said to "channel" a discarnate entity. Whereas a medium relays information from a source that is not physically present, a channeler allows the spirit/entity the temporary use of the physical body in order to convey the information. Such a process has its risks. Throughout history, reports of spirit *possession* consistently suggest that the results are unhealthy for the host. Even in benign cases, however, there can be unintended and unexpected side effects. One man I met many years ago always developed the characteristics of cerebral palsy in his left hand when he channeled. He learned from experience that it was important to have his wife hold his fingers in an open position in order to avoid considerable pain associated with the palsied position of his hand and wrist.

Because of Jenny's prior experience with meditation, she already knew that she had guides available to her. A few weeks after the waking dream presented above, we did some additional hypnosis work in which I utilized her guides more explicitly in the role of co-therapists. I opened this hypnosis work by again reading some comments Angelica had made during an earlier waking dream. I noticed that Jenny flinched at one point.

Therapist: What was that?

Client: I was listening to a talk recently on a CD. One of the messages was "believe in love". The scripturally based talk was living life from the innermost self rather than from the ego. A connection here for me to know is that while the speaker wasn't talking about romantic love because it is limited, there is still an application for romantic love. The application is the same in some way in terms of the fact that the act of living life from the heart—thinking, believing, speaking, doing from the heart—will promote love and will promote a greater possibility of romantic love—the most fulfilling kind—not romantic love, but living from the heart will produce the most fulfilling kind of romantic love. I've listened to that talk thirty times and never associated romantic love with the teaching. [*Pause.*] "Believe in love" has many applications.

Therapist: Did I just see a smile? It looked like the kind of smile that is recognition of a truth.

Client: I've been thinking of giving my boyfriend that talk on CD for his birthday since he asked how to live his life from that place. I think that will be okay to do that.

Therapist: Do you want to check that out? [*Here I am inviting her to check this out at an intuitive level. As you will see below, she checked it out in a different way.*]

Client: Will that be okay to do that? [*Pause.*]

We think that it is fine. [*Notice the shift to using the first-person plural.*]

127

Accompanying the gift it will be good to explain some of the pieces of the talk and help him understand, and give up expectations that he listens to it or understands any of it.

Yup. That's good. [*This is Jenny agreeing with what she just heard.*]

So, it's good for Jenny to remember the virtues that the speaker talks about are ways to experience love: kindness, compassion, generosity, gentleness, etc. [*Notice the shift to referring to Jenny in the third person.*]

Okay. [*Jenny acknowledges what she has just heard.*]

Therapist: Who is "we?"

Client: [*She repeats, "Who is 'we'?"*] We are the ones that help Jenny go about life even when she is not listening.

Therapist: How long have you been working with her?

Client: Many years. We speak to her and she remembers we speak to her as "we" because we've done this work at home.

Therapist: I have a sense that it has not been important for her in the past to know who "we" is.

Client: She's never asked and we have not elaborated as a result.

Therapist: Am I correct that it has not been important?

Client: Correct. The identity is not necessary because there is no form. Identity is important when there is form.

These two sentences have profound implications in our understanding of how life and the universe work! Indeed some of the fascinating research that is currently being done in the field of quantum physics centers on exactly this issue.

Therapist: It would seem, then, that there has been no need for form since she has been able to hear your messages to her simply understanding that they come from "we".

Client: Yes. It would be helpful for her to listen better in moments of anxiety. We did that Thursday night in the meditation after her conversation with [*a friend*] Phil. Sometimes Jenny's mind gets so busy with anxiety that the thoughts in the mind become detrimental and cause the heart to seem less important. So we have to remember a method when this happens.

Therapist: What form [*operant conditioning cue*] might this method take for Jenny?

Client: The form she used this morning when she got anxious. Taking refuge in the mantra, in the breath, in the guru will suffice, and refuge in her friends who know the mantra, the breath, and the guru.

Therapist: Does she need help remembering to remember?

Client: No. [*At this point she spontaneously ended this hypnotic meditation, and uttered the sound of her mantra.*]

In her next session, she got some help from her guides further differentiating how to address the issue of love that is inner-directed. This time, she relayed their thoughts rather than their speaking directly through her.

Client: As an adult I am having to learn that being loved and lovable isn't always going to come from someone or someone loving me every day now. "Now" meaning that as an adult who lives alone and not having been married or in a long-term partnership I have to learn that I'm lovable on my own. When I learn that, when it becomes who I am, then I can attract a mate.

So how do I do that? [*Pause.*] So how do I do that? By offering my feelings of confusion about who I am to God and by giving myself acceptance, compassion, delight. The challenge for me is my will and mind when I make a decision or choice and add my mindfulness to it. My nature is to get stuck there. That can create an obstacle. I am a generous, compassionate, kind-hearted soul and tend to focus that generosity outwardly instead of inwardly as well.

Therapist: I've heard that every time the heart beats, 70 percent of the blood is pumped directly back to the heart muscle. The entire rest of the body only gets 30 percent, yet it seems to function quite well with that ratio. I wonder if you are being invited to shift the ratio of how much love you send to others vs. how much you send to yourself.

Client: I don't know how that is different than what I do. I think it is in compassion, acceptance, and self-love, not so much so in generosity and kindness. Yes, [*she affirms*] compassion, acceptance, and self-love are the qualities to give back to me. [*Then as an aside she says emphatically, "I don't want this struggle anymore!"*]

Therapist: I wonder if your struggle, paradoxically, may have something to do with the effort that it takes to keep trying to direct too much of the heart energy away from yourself.

Client: It is not limited.

Therapist: Is enough coming back?

Client: No. But not because there is not enough to go around. I think I am already ... I think I live my life giving myself those things/ qualities. However, it's because I'm generous with myself that I confuse that with compassion, acceptance, and self-love. I need to understand what compassion, acceptance, and self-love back to me looks like and how it is different than the current reality. That's the question. And the answer is ...?

Therapist: Is there a time from this life when you did this that can serve as an example for you?

Client: When—this is interesting—when my dog died at age 13 my heart hurt so. He got sick when I went to live in the ashram for three months. I left early to take care of him. He died in my arms. Compassion, acceptance, and self-love came in the form of not being critical of myself for leaving him, not making it my fault that he died, and having compassion enough for myself to let myself have another dog so soon afterwards. It was a compassionate response to the sadness.

Therapist: Notice if you can feel the difference and not just be aware of the logical piece of this.

Client: There is contentment. The difference is a deeper contentment. She begins to cry. Okay, so the action and homework will be to inquire about and contemplate compassion towards myself, acceptance and self-love. The action is in the inquiry and can be done daily.

Therapist: I remember Daniel Pinkwater's description of his early days as a writer. He said he committed one hour a day to being

130

available to write. There were days when nothing came out of the pencil onto the paper. There were days when one or two good sentences emerged. There were days when everything he wrote went into the wastebasket.

I suspect that what is important here is the action of the inquiry itself and not the results which come from it. Would you humor me and check with your guides to see if they concur that the critical piece is in the act of inquiry itself as a vehicle for demonstrating compassion, acceptance, and self-love towards yourself?

Client: Yes, it's a step, a big step.

Jenny's exploration of relationships led her to a waking dream that included some unexpected messages from her dream character about suicide. These messages raise interesting spiritual implications, but did not seem to be the focus of the advice that followed from her dream characters and her guides. Rather than experiencing herself as being judged, she was given positive feedback and assistance about how to move forward in her life. If the information she was given is true about the long-term consequences of suicide, it could serve as an important factor for someone who is so depressed as to be considering the option of suicide. Yet independent of the question of reincarnation, the waking dreams seem to have provided Jenny with some constructive suggestions embedded in some emotionally powerful images.

Chapter 12
Putting the Pieces Together

The waking dreams in the previous chapters differ considerably in their specific content, while sharing some common characteristics at a meta-level. In each of the stories, the client became someone else, at times changing gender as the dream character. Whether the person in the dream died of natural causes or because of an accident, following the death there was an experience of floating up out of the body. This was followed by a review of the life of the dream character with a focus on the meaning and interpretation given to certain life events. Then, in various ways, the dream character and the client looked at the implications of this for the client's own life. Despite the sharp, succinct nature of the observations, the client experienced this in a loving, compassionate way. As a therapist, I particularly enjoy how quickly the dream character or the guide seems to zero in on particular beliefs or behaviors that have been problematic for the client.

The process of change in therapy is often accompanied by varying degrees of ambivalence or reluctance. Perhaps because waking dreams are generated internally rather than coming from me in the form of therapeutic metaphors, I find that clients are much more open to taking a good look at themselves. The use of the dream character or guide as a kind of co-therapist fits nicely with this. Clients seem to be able to hear the feedback and advice that they get from the dream character/guide in an open, non-judgmental, non-defensive manner. So following the death of the dream character, I enjoy working together with the dream character/guide to identify and implement new solutions or strategies. As we saw in the story of the caveman, the dream character need not have already died for this process to unfold. We saw a variation of this in Chapter 6 in Eric's waking dream about the drought. Unable to move ahead at the fork in the road of his own life, the client took an interim step in finding strength and compassion to help the dream character face his own, uncertain future.

A single waking dream can help address a specific issue where the client had previously felt stuck. A series of waking dreams does more than allow the client to deal with additional specific issues. Repeat experiences with the NDE-like aspects of the dreams help clients progressively learn how to use these dialogues with dream characters and guides in their daily lives. The most obvious way this occurs is when the client and the dream character establish a cue or signal that will be used to help change a specific behavior. In a broader context, clients learn to recognize and trust their own intuition. There appears to be a considerable parallel between the personal experience of an intuitive moment and the experience of a suggestion or advice from the dream character or a guide. Having found that they can consistently trust the suggestions that they "hear" from their guides, clients seem to increasingly trust their own intuitions.

Trusting intuition becomes even easier as clients notice the differences between intuitive thoughts and fear-based thoughts. Most people have plenty of experience with thoughts based on fear, worry, and anxiety. Such emotions are conspicuously missing in the dialogues clients have with their dream characters and guides. Over a series of waking dreams it becomes easier to recognize internal dialogue that is fear based rather than intuition based. Clients report that they "know" an intuition to be correct. This kind of knowing seems to be associated with an internal sense of calmness, a clear contrast to their fear-based thoughts. Note that this is not to imply that fear does not have any useful purpose. I believe it does. Since fear is always about the unknown, I help clients explore what it is they fear about a particular unknown. Carefully identifying the fear helps transform it into a set of alternative strategies for dealing with the situation.

The wonderfully calm and non-judgmental way in which dream characters and guides help clients deal with current issues also seems to facilitate shifts in attitude. Clients seem progressively better able to approach new situations with greater confidence as this shift takes place. They develop more patience as they allow the time needed for a situation to unfold. Instead of automatically interpreting situations as problems to be "fixed", they increasingly come to see them as containing possibilities for new learning. They also come to know that they are never really alone when confronted with difficult situations. Dorothy experienced this when she was subsequently diagnosed with cancer. She was able to draw on the love and support she had come to know from her dream characters and her guides to help her through the surgery and chemotherapy. The series of waking dreams she had experienced in her therapy had helped further transform her thoughts about death in a way that made it much easier to focus on the opportunities that emerged after her tumor was diagnosed. She remembers being very aware that she was the calmest in the family as she went into surgery.

Waking dreams can occur spontaneously, independent of whether a person is in therapy or not. In addition to the waking dream of my own that I discussed earlier, I have had others that occurred spontaneously, triggered by music. In each case, I returned to the dream content on a number of occasions over a period of months. Just as one can distill multiple layers of meaning by watching a good movie several times, the meaning and transforming power of each of these waking dreams was enhanced each time I revisited them. As has been the case at times for a number of my clients in their own work, both of my own spontaneous waking dreams involved considerable emotional discomfort in the early stages of working with the content. Therefore, it feels prudent to caution the reader that a willingness to explore the depths of one's soul in this manner implies a willingness to experience a variety of emotions with much more intensity than often occurs in daily life. Yet this characteristic of waking dreams is an important part of what gives them their appeal. Perhaps because the life-threatening aspects of a true NDE are predictably absent in waking dreams, and the dream content is arbitrarily defined as fictional, the person is able to enter the experience with a greater trust that whatever happens, he or she will emerge intact.

Most people look forward to experiences that evoke intense "positive" emotions, just as most prefer to forego experiences that evoke intense "negative" emotions. One of the side effects of a series of waking dreams seems to be an increased awareness and tolerance of the idea that being more fully alive requires a willingness to feel emotions more intensely, *regardless* of their valence. The practice acquired while sitting with the intense emotions of waking dreams in the safety of the therapist's office provides a level of assurance that the person can effectively handle this intensity in life outside the office.

Therapists who have experience with hypnosis and related guided imagery tools will likely find it easy to incorporate waking dreams in their work with their clients. It is helpful to have familiarity with the NDE literature to help guide clients who encounter similar kinds of guides. Because the dream content occasionally includes traumatic, albeit fictional, material it is also quite helpful to be familiar with basic trauma treatment strategies. Clients, of course, always have a safety valve: they can stop the dream whenever they choose by simply opening their eyes. For my clients who have trusted the process and the creativity and resourcefulness of their own mind/body/soul, waking dreams have provided a window of opportunity for them to safely experience many of the transforming possibilities of a near-death experience—without the flatline.

My use of waking dreams began pragmatically as one additional tool for helping clients make changes in their lives. Over the years, I sometimes have encountered a client for whom I find I have no solutions to offer despite my love of solving problems. When that happens, I do what most therapists do: I turn to books, articles, and other colleagues to get additional ideas. It was this kind of search that ultimately led me to explore using hypnosis in this way. What I didn't expect when I began using waking dreams were the pro-found, spiritual ripple effects. I do not approach this work with the intent of imposing a particular belief system on my clients. As "real" as the dreams usually seem, I leave the interpretation of them to my clients. Likewise, I do not claim to know who or what the "guides" are that so many of my clients encounter. What I do ask them to notice is how they feel in the presence of them, whether the suggestions they get seem to work, what their intuition tells them about the safety of seeking counsel from their guides. While I would like to say that there has never been an encounter of the spooky kind, I can't. I have had two clients whose dream imagery included beings that they said clearly did not feel safe to them. In both of those situations, I helped them make a quick exit from the scene.

Those who have experienced a true near-death experience typically report major shifts in their spiritual views about the meaning of life and death. Perhaps it is because the after-death experiences in the waking dreams so closely parallel the reports from the NDE literature that clients often find that their own spiritual views begin to change. The differences in the two groups seem to involve the magnitude or pace of the change. The NDE literature suggests that a single such experience is more than adequate to produce major shifts in the person's belief system. Waking dreams seem to work more slowly. I have no satisfactory way to determine if a certain number of waking dreams can or does produce the equivalent effect of a single near-death experience. However, after 19 years of listening to clients describe their own waking dreams, I can say the cumulative effect for me has been quite profound, albeit difficult to articulate.

My clients bring vastly different histories. Some have led relatively peaceful lives and approach therapy not from a place of deficit, but as a pursuit of even higher levels of wellness. Others bring extensive histories of childhood trauma. In order to be fully present in my work with every client, I have found it critical to confront some of my own basic assumptions about the role of God in everyday life. (As this implies, I'm satisfied that God exists. I'm still working on what that means.) It has been important for me to generate some tentative answers to such basic questions as, "How can I believe in a loving God when my 10:30 client who struggles to get by on her monthly disability check was repeatedly raped as a child, and my 2:30 client with the six-figure income comes to do some 'growth work'?" My attempts to put those evolving answers into words have felt quite unsatisfactory. Yet I know that this work has contributed to deep, meaningful changes personally, professionally, and spiritually. A few years ago while having dinner with a colleague who has known me for some 20 years now, I was relating some anecdotes about the impact of this work for me personally. I remarked that years before, one of my own mentors had predicted that one consequence of doing my own work in this area would be that I would laugh more deeply. At the time, I had thought the comment somewhat odd, as I already believed that I had a fairly hearty laugh. I told my colleague, though, that years later I had indeed found this to be true. With a gaze that went right to my core, she quietly remarked, "It's true, you do."

I leave it up to the reader to decide what meaning to attach to the experiences described in these case studies. For myself, what do I make of all this? First, that we are not alone. We are never alone. We are not expected to cope with all of life's challenges without help. I believe every one of us has at least one guide who is available to assist as a mentor, a coach, an adviser. But here's the catch: it seems that our guides are rather limited in the help they can offer unless we specifically ask for it. Fortunately, that part is easy! If you have ever used the Internet to locate information about a topic or a place, you can understand how this works: If you want Google® to do a search for you, *you have to ask for it*. In contrast to the variable quality of the search results on the Internet, however, I find that the help that comes from our guides is of a consistently high quality. There is another advantage. In order to search for something on the Internet, I must be able to connect to an actual website. The help that we get from our guides does not require a conscious two-way connection. In my experience, it is enough to ask for help in one's thoughts.

In the examples presented in this book, clients engaged in two-way conversations with their guides. In day-to-day life, the responses from guides are typically much more subtle. If you have asked your guide to give you a hand on a particular matter, you may find yourself beginning to experience one or more of a series of "coincidences". A phrase or a sentence may suddenly stand out for you in a very timely way. In the midst of wrestling with a difficult issue or a dark mood, you may find that the lyrics of a song you have heard many times in the past suddenly speak to you in a very personal way. A friend may tell you about a book she has been reading that offers you new insights about some issue that you had been confronting.

However we understand the journey of the soul across this lifetime or across many lifetimes, I have continued to find great comfort in the profound love and support that my own guides have offered me. Whether a particular waking dream is just good fiction generated by a person's mind motivated by a wish for wellness, or whether the imagery is really that of memories from another lifetime, is a moot point from a pragmatic clinical perspective. The NDE-like aspects of the experience provide a rich catalyst for personal transformation that transcends the boundaries and severe limitations of language.

When I began exploring the use of waking dreams as a tool for helping people change, not much was being written about the intersection between science and spirituality. In the years since then, there has been a significant shift in public perception where spirituality is concerned that is slowly rippling into the professional community. Not only have there been a number of books, movies, and TV shows that have incorporated metaphysical content, but professional journals, books, and conferences are becoming increasingly open to the exploration of these topics. As the experiences in this book have done for me, I offer them to you in the hope that they will similarly fuel your curiosity about life beyond the illusory confines of three-dimensional space and time and your true awe and wonder of that which remains unknown and mysterious the further that your own explorations carry you.

Bibliography

Almeder, Robert (1987). *Beyond Death*, Chicago, Charles C. Thomas.

Almeder, Robert (1992). *Death and Personal Survival: Evidence for Life after Death*, Lanham, MD, Littlefield Adams Quality Paperbacks.

Bache, Christopher (1991). *Lifecycles: Reincarnation and the Web of Life*, St. Paul, MN, Paragon House.

Borysenko, Joan (1987). *Minding the Body, Mending the Mind*, Reading, MA, Addison-Wesley.

Cardena, Etzel, Steven Lynn and Stanley Krippner (eds) (2000). *Varieties of Anomalous Experience: Examining the Scientific Evidence*, Washington, D.C., American Psychological Association.

Ducasse, C.J. (1961). *A Critical Examination of the Belief in a Life after Death*, Chicago, Charles C. Thomas.

Gershom, Yonassan (1992). *Beyond the Ashes: Cases of Reincarnation from the Holocaust*, Virginia Beach, VA, A.R.E. Press.

Grof, Stan (1985). *Beyond the Brain*, Albany, NY, State University of New York Press.

Kelly, G. (1963). *A Theory of Personality*, NY, W.W. Norton.

Lucas, Winafred Blake (1993). *Regression Therapy: A Handbook for Professionals, Vol. 1: Past-Life Therapy; Vol. 2: Special Instances of Altered State Work*, Crest Park, CA, Deep Forest Press.

Mehl-Madrona and Andrew Weil (1997). *Coyote Medicine: Lessons from Native American Healing*, NY, Fireside.

Moody, Raymond (1975). *Life After Life*, Aptos, CA, Mockingbird Press.

Moody, Raymond (1991). *Coming Back: A Psychiatrist Explores Past-Life Journeys*, NY, Bantam.

Moody, Raymond (1999). *The Last Laugh*, Charlottesville, VA, Hampton Roads.

Myss, Caroline (1996). *Anatomy of the Spirit: The Seven Stages of Power and Healing*, NY, Harmony Books.

Ring, Kenneth (1985). *Heading Toward Omega: In Search of the Meaning of the Near-Death Experience*, NY, William Morrow.

Ring, Kenneth and Sharon Cooper (1999). *Mindsight: Near-Death and Out-of-Body Experiences in the Blind*, Palo Alto, CA, William James Center for Consciousness Studies.

Rommer, Barbara (2000). *Blessing in Disguise: Another Side of the Near-death Experience*, St. Paul, MN, Llewellyn Publications.

Rossi, Ernest (1988). *The Psychobiology of Mind-Body Healing: New Concepts of Therapeutic Hypnosis*, NY, W.W. Norton.

Rossi, Ernest and David Cheek (1988). *Mind-Body Therapy: Methods of Ideodynamic Healing in Hypnosis*, NY, W.W. Norton.

Sabom, Michael B. (1982). *Recollections of Death: A Medical Investigation*, NY, Simon & Schuster.

Sabom, Michael (1998). *Light & Death: One Doctor's Fascinating Account of Near-death Experiences*, Grand Rapids, MI, Zondervan.

Sacerdote, Paul (1967). *Induced Dreams: About the Theory and Therapeutic Applications of Dreams Hypnotically Induced*, NY, Theo Gaus, Ltd.

Schwartz, Gary, and William Simon (2002). *The Afterlife Experiments: Breakthrough Scientific Evidence of Life After Death*, NY, Pocket Books.

Schwartz, Gary, and Linda Russek (1999). *The Living Energy Universe*, Charlottesville, VA, Hampton Roads.

Stevenson, Ian (1987). *Children Who Remember Previous Lives: A Question of Reincarnation*, Charlottesville, VA, University Press of Virginia.

Stevenson, Ian (1997). *Reincarnation and Biology: A Contribution to the Etiology of Birthmarks and Birth Defects, Vols 1* and 2, Westport, CT, Praeger.

Stevenson, Ian (1997). *Where Reincarnation and Biology Intersect*, Westport, CT, Praeger.

Talbot, Michael (1991). *Holographic Universe*, NY, HarperCollins.

Ten Dam, Hans (1996). *Deep Healing: A Practical Guide of Past-Life Therapy, Amsterdam*, Netherlands, Tasso.

Weiss, Brian (1988). *Many Lives, Many Masters*, NY, Simon & Schuster.

Weiss, Brian (1992). *Through Time into Healing*, NY, Simon & Schuster.

Weiss, Brian (1996). *Only Love is Real: A Story of Soulmates Reunited*, NY, Warner Books.

Weiss, Brian (2000). *Messages From the Masters: Tapping into the Power of Love*, NY, Warner Books.

Wilber, Ken (1985). *The Spectrum of Consciousness*, Wheaton, IL, Theosophical (Quest Books).

Zukav, Gary (1979). *The Dancing Wi-Li Masters*, NY, Morrow.

Zukav, Gary (1999). *Seat of the Soul*, NY, Simon & Schuster.

Endnotes

1. Peterson, R. (1997). *Out of Body Experiences: How to Have Them and What to Expect*, Charlottesville, VA: Hampton Roads Publishing Co., pp. 8–9.

2. Borysenko, Joan (1997). *The Ways of the Mystic: Seven Paths to God*, Carlsbad, CA: Hay House, Inc., pp. xi–xii.

3. Borysenko, Joan (1997), pp. 8–9.

4. Weiss, Brian (1988). *Many Lives, Many Masters*, NY: Simon & Schuster.

5. Lucas, W.B., (ed.) (1993). *Regression Therapy: A Handbook for Professionals: Volume I: Past-Life Therapy*, Visalia, CA: Jostens Press, p. 4.

6. Denning, H.M. in Lucas, W.B. editor, (1993). *Regression Therapy: A Handbook for Professionals: Volume I: Past-Life Therapy*, Visalia, CA: Jostens Press, p. 196.

Index